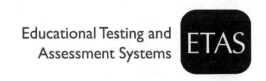

Educational Testing and
Assessment Systems ETAS

INTERNAL MEDICINE IN-REVIEW
STUDY GUIDE

MODULE 1

Companion to the Online Study System
InReviewIM.com

Senior Editor
Norman H. Ertel, MD

Associate Editors
James M. Horowitz, MD
Miguel A. Paniagua, MD, FACP

*Available through support
from the makers of*

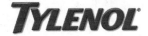

Powered by

Castle Connolly Graduate
Medical Publishing

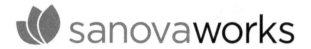

ISBN 978-0-9858025-1-6

© 2012 Published by Educational Testing & Assessment Systems, a product of SanovaWorks
Edited by Norman H. Ertel, MD

Printed in the United States of America

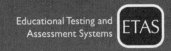
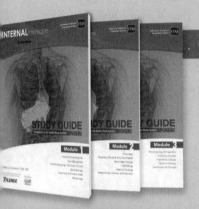
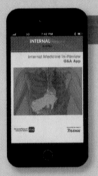
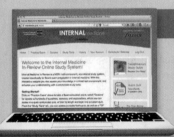
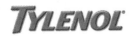

LETTER FROM THE EDITOR

Dear Colleague,

With great pleasure we present to you the the inaugural edition of the Internal Medicine In-Review Study Guide, developed and published by Educational Testing and Assessment Systems (ETAS) in collaboration with Castle Connolly Graduate Medical Publishing (CCGMP).

Authored by over 20 leading academic faculty from various fields, the contributing authors have created a study guide that covers the core topics that are found on the American Board of Internal Medicine certification examination blueprint.

Our goal is to provide you with comprehensive yet high-yield information in a user-friendly format to help make your study for the Board exam both efficient and streamlined. In our attempt to meet this aim, and in light of resident and educator feedback, we have fashioned a multi-modal program, which includes the comprehensive written text, presented in a three-module booklet set, an interactive online study system (InReviewIM.com), and a Q&A smartphone app. Together these tools provide relevant information and methods to prepare you for your exams.

You will also note a pain management chapter in this study guide, which is not expressly identified as a content area covered on the ABIM certification exam; however, pain management can be found throughout many of the medical-content categories, including the 3% of the exam referred to as "Miscellaneous." Beyond exam study, we firmly believe that pain management knowledge is crucially important for healthcare providers in their day-to-day practice.

The makers of TYLENOL® have generously provided the support needed to make this program available to US-based internal medicine residents at no cost. We are grateful for their commitment to education.

Finally, as part of our ongoing efforts to refine the Internal Medicine In-Review program, we encourage you to provide feedback on the study guide. Any comments or suggestions you have will help to ensure that we create an educational tool that meets residents' needs and is even more useful in the years to come.

We wish you the best of luck in your studies and on the Board!

Sincerely,

Norman H. Ertel, MD and the Internal Medicine In-Review Team

F A C U L T Y

Senior Editor

Norman H. Ertel, MD
Professor of Medicine, Emeritus
University of Medicine and Dentistry of
New Jersey
Newark, NJ

Associate Editors

James M. Horowitz, MD
Chief Resident
New York Presbyterian Hospital - Weill Cornell
Medical Center
Department of Medicine
New York, NY

Miguel A. Paniagua, MD, FACP
Associate Professor, Department of
Internal Medicine
Director, Internal Medicine Residency
Training Programs
Saint Louis University School of
Medicine Program
Department of Internal Medicine
Saint Louis, MO

Authors

Jastin Antisdel, MD
Assistant Professor
Director, Rhinology and Sinus Surgery
Saint Louis University School of Medicine
Saint Louis, MO

Sarah Boutwell, MD
Saint Louis University School of Medicine
Department of Internal Medicine
Saint Louis, MO

Fred Buckhold, MD
Assistant Professor, Division of General
Internal Medicine
Associate Program Directory, Internal
Medicine Residency
Saint Louis University School of Medicine
Department of Internal Medicine
Saint Louis, MO

Elie Chahla, MD
Assistant Professor
Saint Louis University School of Medicine
Department of Internal Medicine
Saint Louis, MO

Luis Chaves, MD
Chief Resident, Adult Psychiatry Program
University of Miami - Miller School of
Medicine Department of Psychiatry and
Behavioral Sciences
Miami, FL

Harvey Chitiva, MD
Fellow, Child/Adolescent Program
University of Miami - Miller School of
Medicine Department of Psychiatry and
Behavioral Sciences
Miami, FL

FACULTY

Dary J. Costa, MD
Assistant Professor, Pediatric Otolaryngology
Cardinal Glennon Children's Medical Center
Saint Louis, MO

Matthew D. Council, MD
Assistant Professor
Saint Louis Unveristy - Saint Louis Eye Institute
Saint Louis, MO

Cheston Cunha, MD
Fellow
Brown University - Alpert School of Medicine
Division of Infectious Diseases
Providence, RI

Anne Davis, MD
Assistant Clinical Professor of Obstetrics and
Gynecology
Columbia University Medical Center
New York, NY

Wasseem El-Aneed, MD
Saint Louis University School of Medicine
Department of Internal Medicine
Saint Louis, MO

Deepika Fernandes, MD
Saint Louis University School of Medicine
Department of Internal Medicine
Saint Louis, MO

Adam Friedman, MD, FAAD
Instructor, Director of Dermatology Research,
Associate Residency Program Director
Albert Einstein College of Medicine
Division of Dermatology
Bronx, NY

Mustafa Hyder, MD
Saint Louis University School of Medicine
Department of Internal Medicine
Saint Louis, MO

Edward Kessler, MD
Saint Louis University School of Medicine
Department of Internal Medicine
Saint Louis, MO

Matthew J. Mandel, MD
Board Certified Neurologist
Cambridge, MA

Saakshi Khattri, MD
Fellow
Albert Einstein College of Medicine
Division of Rheumatology
Bronx, NY

Kathleen Molly McShane, MD, MPH
Assistant Professor
University of Miami - Miller School of
Medicine Department of Psychiatry and
Behavioral Sciences
Miami, FL

Genevieve Moyer, MD
Saint Louis University School of Medicine
Department of Internal Medicine
Saint Louis, MO

Lorraine L. Rosamilia, MD, FAAD
Staff Physician
Geisinger Health System Department
of Dermatology
State College, PA

Michael Sanley, MD
Chief Resident, Clinical Instructor
Saint Louis University School of Medicine
Department of Internal Medicine
Saint Louis, MO

F A C U L T Y

Radu V. Saveanu, MD
Vice Chair for Education
Director, Psychiatry Residency Training Program
University of Miami - Miller School of Medicine
Department of Psychiatry and Behavioral
Sciences
Miami, FL

Mohamed Abou Shousha, MD
Saint Louis Unveristy - Saint Louis Eye Institute
Saint Louis, MO

Plinio P. Silva, MD, MPH
House Staff
Albany Medical Center
Department of Anesthesiology
Albany, NY

Howard S. Smith, MD
Professor of Anesthesiology, Internal Medicine,
and Physical Medicine and Rehabiliation
Albany Medical Center
Department of Anesthesiology
Albany, NY

Alexandra Voinescu, MD
Assistant Professor of Internal Medicine/
Nephrology
Saint Louis University School of Medicine
Division of Nephrology
Saint Louis, MO

Yashaswini Yeragunta, MD
Saint Louis University School of Medicine
Department of Internal Medicine
Saint Louis, MO

Ashraf Qaqa, MD
Fellow
Seton Hall University - St. Michael's Medical
Center - School of Health and Medical Sciences
Department of Cardiology
Newark, NJ

Chief Resident Feedback Group

Katayoun Edalat Parsi, MS, DO
2012/2013 Chief Resident
University of California San Francisco, Fresno
Medical Education Program
Fresno, CA

Marcus A. Crosby, MD
2012/2013 Chief Resident
Gundersen Lutheran Medical Foundation
La Crosse, WI

Shahrod Mokhtari, MD
2012/2013 Chief Resident
University of Southern California
LAC + USC Medical Center
Los Angeles, CA

Special Recognition

Farid Razavi, MD
New York Presbyterian-Weill Cornell
Department of Medicine
New York, NY

MODULE 1 - CONTENTS

MODULE 1 - CONTENTS

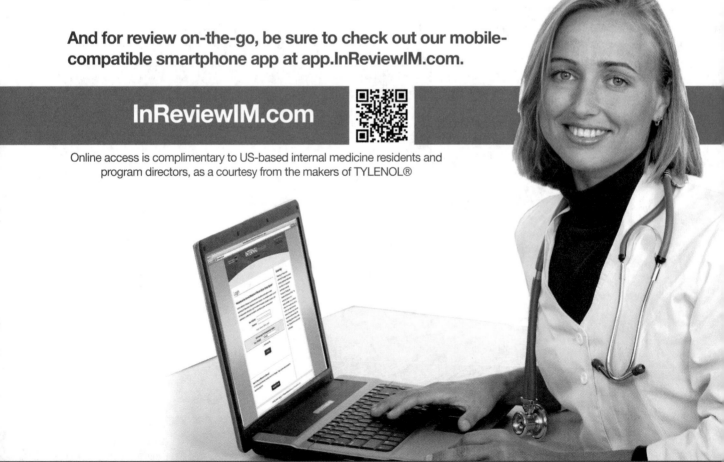
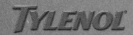

1 General Internal Medicine

Fred Buckhold, MD

Contents

1.1 ROUTINE CARE OF THE HEALTHY PATIENT

Screening

Assessing patients for risk or presence of asymptomatic disease and identifying lifestyle choices that have health consequences.

- Often based on prevalence of diseases
- The United States Preventative Services Task Force (USPSTF) has recommendations on which screening measures are effective

Screening During History and Physical Exam

- Measure height and weight (for BMI/obesity)
- Measure blood pressure (for hypertension)
- Assess for tobacco, alcohol, and drug use
- Detailed sexual history, including risk factors for STDs

Screening Tests

- Papanicolaou test every 3 years starting at age 21, stopping age 65
- Chlamydia for sexually active women under age of 25
- Routine HIV screening for ages 13 to 64
- Biennial mammograms for women age 50 to 74
- Cholesterol screening (Total and HDL) every 5 years in men >35 years and women >45 years
- Fasting glucose if sustained blood pressure >135/80 mmHg
- Colonoscopy every 10 years above age of 50 until age 74; may also have occult blood testing yearly or flexible sigmoidoscopy every 5 years
- Abdominal aortic aneurysm for male adults between 65 to 75, if history of smoking present
- Osteoporosis (via BMD) in women >65, or 60 to 64 if body weight below 70 kg

Family History

Taking a Family History

- Screen for diseases that family members have
- Inquire specifically about early onset cardiovascular disease and 1st and 2nd degree relatives with cancer (and what type/age of onset)

Genetic Testing

- More useful for high risk populations, or if suspected
- Testing should aid in diagnosis and/or management
  - BRCA or FAP mutation may lead to aggressive screening and interventions

Immunizations

Table 1.1: Immunizations

Vaccine	Frequency	Indications (blank indicates universal)
Hepatitis A	2 doses once	• Men who have sex with men • Injection drug users • Occupational (food handlers) • Travel to endemic areas • Chronic liver disease
Hepatitis B	3 doses	• Sexually active young adults • Healthcare or public safety workers • Travel
Human papillomavirus vaccine	Females 19-26 years, males 19-21 years, consider 22-26 – 3 doses	
Influenza	Annually	
Measles-Mumps-Rubella	Should have as a child	May have to check serologies if unsure of history; adults born before 1957 considered immune
Meningococcal vaccine	1 dose	• 1st year college students • HIV or asplenia
Pneumococcal vaccine	1 or 2 doses	• Age >65 • Chronic lung disease, diabetes, chronic liver disease, asplenia
Tetanus-Diphtheria-Acellular Pertussis (Td or Tdap)	Every 10 years	• Tdap booster once, followed by Td every 10 years
Varicella	2 doses	
Zoster	1 dose	Age 60 and above

Lifestyle Risk Factors

Behavioral Counseling
- Brief interventions at office visits can be effective
- Use the 5 "A"s: **A**ssess, **A**dvise, **A**gree, **A**ssist, **A**rrange

Physical Inactivity
- Should encourage 30 minutes of aerobic exercise 5 times weekly
- Strengthening exercise at least twice weekly
- Medical screening not needed in asymptomatic patients
- Encourage activity to reduce sedentary behavior for those with chronic disease or in ages >65 years

Substance Use Disorders
- Tobacco
  - Assess at each visit
  - Brief counseling and possibly medication
- Routinely screen for alcohol misuse and abuse—most frequently in young adults and smokers
  - Can use CAGE questionnaire

- If at-risk—brief counseling
- If dependence—referral to treatment
- Illicit drugs: Look for behavior changes, legal troubles, and medical sequelae
  - Referral or brief counseling

Sexual Behavior
- History oriented to high risk practices (men who have sex with men, multiple partners, contact with sex workers)
- Counsel of safe sex practices (use of barrier protection vs. birth control for prevention of STDs)
- Offer screening for STDs as appropriate

Domestic Violence
- Screen if suspected
- Intervene if possible; assessing for safety, clear documentation of injuries, and providing resources

1.2 GERIATRIC MEDICINE

Functional Assessment
- Hearing loss screening
  - Patient reported
  - Test by whispering in ear while using distraction in other ear
- Screen for vision loss
- Screen for depression
- Probe for deficits in activities of daily living
- Inquire for falls
  - "Get up and go" good for screening
  - To reduce risk of falls:
    - Monitor meds, stop centrally acting ones
    - Muscle strengthening and balance exercises
    - Calcium and vitamin D
    - Improve living environment

Urinary Incontinence
- Stress: Loss of sphincter tone, worse with cough
  - Pelvic floor exercises
  - Estrogen cream
  - Surgery
- Urge: Spastic/overactive detrusor muscle
  - Timed voiding
  - Anticholinergics
- In men: Consider overflow incontinence from bladder retention from BPH

Pressure Ulcers
Prevent them at all costs, aimed at reducing friction, shear stress, and skin moisture.
- May need debridement and antibiotics for stage III-IV ulcers

1.3 PERI-OPERATIVE MEDICINE

There are few limiting factors that would prevent a patient from being an operative candidate. Evaluation goal is risk reduction if possible, and perform testing only if it will change pre-operative management.

Cardiac Evaluation

- ACC/AHA algorithm
    1. Emergent surgery → to OR
    2. Active cardiac condition (ACS, ventricular arrhythmia, decompensated heart failure) → treat condition
    3. Low risk surgery → to OR
    4. Assess functional capacity (can walk up a flight of stairs or hill → go to OR)
    5. If unable to assess or perform at functional capacity, assess risk factors; if 3 or more consider testing if it will change management
- Risk factors
    ◦ High risk surgery
    ◦ Creatinine >2.0
    ◦ Ischemic heart disease
    ◦ History of stroke
    ◦ Diabetes requiring insulin
    ◦ LV systolic dysfunction with EF <35%
- If patient has coronary revascularization prior to surgery (either due to pre-operative assessment or not), needs to be on anti-platelet agents for 4 to 6 weeks for bare metal stent, 12 months for drug eluting stent
    ◦ Both aspirin and clopidogrel should be stopped about 5 days before planned surgery
- Maintain β-blocker dose if already taking—no need to add before surgery
- Consider stopping lisinopril

Pulmonary Evaluation

- Risk factors associated with pulmonary complications
    ◦ Type of surgery (emergent vs. non-emergent) and surgery duration
    ◦ Location (intrathoracic and upper abdominal highest risk)
    ◦ Use of general anesthesia, long acting neuromuscular blockers, and NG tubes
- Only measure to reduce morbidity/mortality is incentive spirometry postoperatively
- Only do diagnostic spirometry pre-operatively if having lung resection
    ◦ Chest radiograph not needed

VTE Prophylaxis

- Should be applied to most surgical patients (mechanical and pharmacologic)
    ◦ Usually LMWH or heparin is sufficient
    ◦ Higher risk surgeries (hip or knee arthroplasty, hip fracture, trauma, spinal injury): Therapeutic warfarin for INR 2-3 or fondaparinux

Glycemic Control

- Diabetics should be monitored closely peri-operatively
- Data unclear on optimal regimen, likely benefit if blood sugar remains less than 180 mg/dL
    ◦ Continue insulin regimen (basal, no bolus) for type 1 diabetics

- Halve insulin for type 2 diabetics the day of surgery
- Metformin and other agents should be stopped 1 to 3 days prior to operation

Other Considerations
- Surgery in a hyperthyroid patient may induce thyroid storm
  - May use steroids to block this effect
- Stress steroids may be required for steroid-dependent patients
- Dialysis patients should ideally be dialyzed the day prior to surgery
- Delirium commonly occurs in patients at risk

1.4 PATIENT SAFETY
- Data on adverse events
  - IOM report (To Err is Human) – 100,000 deaths annually from medical error
  - Majority are medication related
- Principles of patient safety
  - Root cause analysis to define cause
  - Redundancy in system
  - Checklists
  - "Time-outs"
  - Electronic medical records
- Quality improvement models
  - Most common – PDSA; **P**lan – **D**o – **S**tudy – **A**ct
  - 6 sigma
  - Total quality management
- Diagnostic error
  - Heuristics (mental shortcuts) lead to diagnostic mistakes
    - Availability
    - Anchoring
    - Blind obedience
  - Can be reduced by recognizing types of heuristics, completeness of differential diagnosis, and by considering alternative diagnosis along with working diagnosis
- National Patient Safety Goals
  - Mandated by Joint Commission in 2009
    - Emphasize areas of risk in patient care, including medication safety, patient hand-offs, infection control

1.5 PROFESSIONALISM AND ETHICS
- Professionalism – 3 principles from the Charter of Medical Professionalism
  - Primacy of patient welfare
  - Patient autonomy
  - Social justice
- Assessing decision-making capacity
  - Does the patient have the ability (medical or psychological) to make decisions
  - Multiple modalities based on stringency – best tests find rationality in choice
    - "Why are you choosing this?"

- Does the decision make sense?
- Advance directives and surrogate decision-making
  - Advance directives – instructions on types of care to be provided. May be vague
  - Surrogate decision maker – healthcare proxy or power of attorney; typically a family member
    - Makes decisions on behalf of patient with patient's known preferences in mind
- Informed consent – 3 elements
  - Disclosure of all relevant information – benefits, risks, alternatives – within reason
  - Adequate understanding by the patient
  - Voluntary decision
- Withholding or withdrawing care
  - Justifiable if futile
  - Ideally should be discussed with patient as early as possible
  - Should try to involve family and patient as much as possible
- Physician-assisted suicide and euthanasia
  - Physician-assisted suicide illegal except in Washington and Oregon
  - Euthanasia (physician directly administering a substance causing death) is illegal
  - Patient inquiries should be a means to assessing need for care
- Confidentiality
  - Strive to maintain at all costs; consent must be obtained to release patient health information
- Conflicts of interest
  - Occurs when other interests to provider may potentially or does interfere with provider's duty to patient
  - Can be handled by:
    - Disclosure – making conflict known
    - Avoidance – avoiding conflict
- Medical error reporting
  - When error occurs – inform patient
- Sexual contact between physician and patient is unethical, even with former patients
- The impaired physician and colleague responsibility
  - Ethical responsibility to report suspected impairment

1.6 PALLIATIVE CARE

Assessment
- Center around terminal diagnosis, expected symptoms, and ways to alleviate symptoms
- Performance scales aid in prognosis
- Consider stopping medical devices

Symptom Management
- Pain: Aspirin, acetaminophen, or NSAIDs initially, at labeled dosing. For severe pain, opioids are reasonable
  - Can use combination regimen of long acting and short acting opioids
  - Oral is preferred, avoid meperidine and opioid agonists/antagonists
  - Liquid morphine may be helpful for those with difficulty swallowing

- Monitor for side effects
- Surgery may be useful for visceral pain
- Appropriate agents for neuropathic pain include TCAs, dual acting anti-depressants, tramadol, gabapentin, pregabalin
- Dyspnea: Treat the symptom
  - Use short acting opioid if on chronic therapy for symptom relief
  - Morphine also helpful
  - Do not use benzodiazepines
  - Oxygen for hypoxemia
- Nutrition: Appetite may wane, but important to consider social element of eating
  - If not near death, stimulants are appropriate - megestrol and medroxyprogesterone
  - Unclear benefit of enteral/parental feeding
- Depression: Difficult to diagnose
  - Patients noting low mood and low interest are more likely to be depressed
  - Treat with SSRIs or TCAs
- Altered mental status
  - Consider medication, especially opioids
  - Consider prognosis before full evaluation
  - Haloperidol may be used for symptoms, can also use benzodiazepine with monitoring
- Caregiver stressors and bereavement
  - Must be closely monitored
  - If symptoms of bereavement continue for 6 months, high risk for complicated grief and depression – may need treatment medically or with therapy

1.7 COMMON SYMPTOMS

Chronic Pain
- Characterizing and assessing pain
  - Somatic pain: Inflammatory, responds to NSAIDs
  - Central sensitization pain – abnormal processing of sensation by CNS; allodynia and hyperalgesia is common
    - Opioids and NSAIDs often not helpful
    - Cognitive therapy, serotonin-norepinephrine reuptake inhibitors, and TCAs are helpful
  - Evaluate and treat comorbid depression and anxiety
  - If history or physical suggest possible etiology for pain, evaluate with appropriate tests, otherwise none is needed
- Managing pain
  - The World Health Organization's Analgesic Ladder is a useful construct
    - Start with non-opioids (NSAIDs, aspirin, acetaminophen), before starting mild opioids (codeine), followed by strong opioids (morphine, fentanyl) with careful consideration of side effects and potential for abuse
    - Liquid morphine effective for those with difficulty swallowing
    - Tramadol is an effective alternative

- Non-pharmacologic
  - Ice for inflammatory pain
  - Heat for chronic pain
  - Graded exercise
  - Electrical nerve stimulation

Acute and Chronic Cough

- Acute (less than 3 weeks) – commonly:
  - Usually infectious, use other clues for diagnosis
    - Viral URI
    - Viral or bacterial pneumonia – unlikely unless abnormal vital signs (fever, HR >100 BPM, respirations >24/min) or physical exam findings
    - Bacterial sinusitis – 7 days or more of symptoms
    - Rhinitis with post-nasal drip
    - Acute bronchitis – non-productive cough, likely viral, symptomatic care
    - Influenza – if in season (fall/winter), concomitant fever, malaise, cough, sore throat
- Chronic (more than 8 weeks) or sub-acute (3 to 8 weeks). Most commonly:
  - Asthma – confirmed when improved with asthma treatment
  - GERD – therapeutic trial with PPI is reasonable
  - Post nasal drip/upper airway cough syndrome
    - If cause unclear, 1st step is empiric therapy with antihistamine/decongestant
  - Alternative diagnoses
    - ACE inhibitor
    - Chronic bronchitis (if sputum production)
    - Non-asthmatic eosinophilic bronchitis
    - Smoking (improves with cessation)
- Cough in the immunocompromised patient
  - Consider opportunistic infections, tuberculosis, and pneumocystis pneumonia
- Hemoptysis
  - Malignancy, infection, elevated pulmonary pressure, or idiopathic
  - Should have chest X-ray
    - If male, older than 40 years, symptoms >1 week, or 40 pack year smoker – chest CT and bronchoscopy
  - If massive bleeding needs emergent/critical care

Chronic Fatigue and Chronic Fatigue Syndrome

- Defined as disabling fatigue lasting more than 6 months
- Etiology unknown
- Rule out other factors (OSA or other sleep disturbance, depression, anemia, drugs, hypothyroid, chronic disease)
- Cognitive behavioral therapy and graded exercise are effective therapies
- Antidepressants might be helpful

Dizziness

- Helpful exam maneuvers
  - Orthostatics for lightheadedness
  - Dix-Hallpike for positional vertigo
  - Neurologic and ear assessment for vertigo

Vestibular and Peripheral Nerve Causes of Dizziness
- Usually related to vertigo
  - BPPV – use Epley maneuver to improve
  - Vestibular neuronitis – likely after viral infection; symptoms not self limiting
    - May respond to steroids
  - Meniere – vertigo with hearing loss and tinnitus
    - Thiazide diuretics to treat

Central Nervous System Causes of Dizziness
- Rarely tumor
- Vascular disease of posterior cerebral arteries; consider when other vascular risk factors present
- Migraine headaches
- MRI may be helpful if symptoms or exam suggest

Disequilibrium – Gait Unsteadiness
- Multifactorial – peripheral neuropathy, poor eyesight, medications
- Safety features added to homes, assistive devices, and reducing polypharmacy helpful

Non-specific Dizziness
- May be related to other systemic problems (hypoglycemia, hyperventilation)
- Associated with psychiatric illness

Insomnia
- Often related to co-morbidities
- Take a detailed history involving time going to sleep, duration, wakefulness upon waking
- Non-drug therapies (sleep restriction, cognitive therapy, sleep journal) likely more effective than drug therapies
- Can use medication, preferably not benzodiazepines

Syncope
Transient loss of consciousness due to lack of cerebral blood flow. *Pre-syncope* is the sensation of almost losing consciousness. Pathophysiology typically the same for both.

Table 1.2: Syncope

Etiology/Cause of Syncope	Clues
Vasovagal	• Symptoms occur after sudden pain, fear, or unpleasant sensation • After prolonged standing
Situational	Based on history
Carotid-sinus	Occurs with head rotation or palpation of carotid sinus
Psychiatric disorders	• Somatic symptoms, high frequency of occurrences • Associated with anxiety, depression, panic disorder
Orthostatic hypotension	Occurs when standing from supine/sitting
Medication	Consider when polypharmacy, many centrally acting drugs, or that affect QT interval
Neurologic (stroke, seizure, etc.)	• Migraines • Symptoms suggestive of posterior stroke • Seizure
Structural heart disease (outflow obstruction or ischemia)	• Atrial myxoma or thrombus – symptoms with positional changes, no orthostasis • Exertional symptoms – structural changes in heart (AS, MS, HOCM)
Arrhythmia	• Brief LOC with no prodrome • Family history of sudden death
Idiopathic	Other causes ruled out

Adapted from Kapoor W, NEJM 343:1856-62.

- Patients with high index of suspicion for heat disease (based on previous history or ECG changes) should be admitted for evaluation
- Evaluation should be based on suspected underlying condition

Chest Pain

- Priority in differential diagnosis depends on situation
  - Majority of CP in ambulatory clinic – musculoskeletal
  - In emergency settings – acute coronary syndrome
- Differential is broad; clues to diagnosis include:
  - Ischemic changes to heart: Substernal pain or tightness with radiation; ECG and biochemical changes
    - Reproducible, sharp pain, negative ECG, or positional-related makes ischemia unlikely
  - Aortic dissection – abrupt onset, tearing chest pain, pulse differential, wide mediastinum on chest X-ray – if considering, order MRI, angiography, or chest CT (not echo)
  - Pulmonary embolism – pleuritic pain, sudden onset, dyspnea, tachycardia, and risk factors; CT angio is reasonable if intermediate or high suspicion
  - Pneumonia – fever, productive cough, infiltrate on chest X-ray
  - Gastroesophageal reflux – often mimics ischemic heart disease, always consider cardiac disease. Trial of proton pump inhibitor if cardiac disease ruled out
  - Musculoskeletal – reproducible tenderness, otherwise normal exam
  - Panic attack or anxiety

Hyperlipidemia

- Screening – males >35, females >45
- Components of cholesterol profile
  - LDL – main substrate for atherogenic disease. Usually elevated due to dietary/lifestyle or genetic causes, also consider hypothyroidism, nephrotic syndrome, obstructive liver disease, and certain medications
    - Primary target of cholesterol lowering therapy
  - Triglycerides – not reliable predictor of cardiovascular disease; if high, may affect estimation of LDL (LDL not usually measured directly)
    - Must treat if above 500 mg/dL to decrease risk of pancreatitis
  - HDL – higher levels correlate with decreased incidence of cardiovascular disease; no evidence that raising improves CAD risk
- Treatment
  - Lifestyle modifications 1st choice – restriction of fat, more plant stenosis, exercise
  - Statins are mainstay of secondary prevention (for those who have CAD), and should be considered for primary prevention if risk is high enough
    - Must be vigilant for effects of myopathy and myalgia, elevated liver enzymes, and rhabdomyolysis
  - Other drugs – fibrates (mainly gemfibrozil), ezetimibe, and niacin may be used to further reduce LDL or improve HDL, but benefit on atherogenic disease is uncertain
  - Goals to treat with medication
    - Use Framingham Risk Score (FRS) to assess 10 year cardiovascular risk
    - Risk factors for CVD
      - Cigarette smoking
      - Hypertension
      - Age (men ≥45, women ≥55)
      - Low HDL (<40 mg/dl)
      - Family history – male relative with CAD <55, female <65
    - If CVD present, treat LDL ≥100 mg/dL
    - If FRS 10 to 20%, ≥2 risk factors, treat if LDL ≥130 mg/dL
    - If FRS <10%, ≥2 risk factors, treat LDL ≥160 mg/dL
    - If FRS <10%, 0 to 1 risk factors, treat LDL ≥190 mg/dL
    - If LDL is lower than above numbers, but elevated, start lifestyle changes

Obesity

- Defined as BMI >30
- Obesity confers higher risk of chronic disease
- Evaluation should probe for causes, including:
  - Medication induced
  - Endocrine – hypothyroid, excess cortisol, polycystic ovarian syndrome
  - Other cardiovascular comorbidities (hypertension, diabetes, dyslipidemia)
- Treatment
  - Diet and exercise
  - Behavior modification
  - Orlistat and sibutramine can be used as supplement to above
    - Sibutramine should not be used in hypertensive patients

- Bariatric surgery has been shown to reduce incidence of diabetes, hypertension, sleep apnea, and hyperlipidemia
  - Monitor long term for nutrient deficiencies, especially vitamin B12, vitamin D, calcium, iron, folate

1.8 MEN'S HEALTH

- Erectile dysfunction is often due to organic factors similar to cardiovascular disease (smoking, hypertension, and diabetes)
  - Try to identify comorbid disease
  - Treat initially with phosphodiesterase -5 inhibitors, if no contraindications (i.e., not on nitrates)
- Premature ejaculation – treat with SSRIs or behavioral techniques
- Decreased libido
  - Hormone defect (testosterone or hyperprolactinemia)
  - Psychiatric illness (depression)
  - Medications
- Benign prostatic hyperplasia (BPH)
  - Enlargement of prostate causing obstruction of urine flow – can lead to overflow incontinence
  - Large, boggy prostate on exam
  - Consider mitigating factors – fluid ingestion, medications, neurologic/cognitive impairments
  - Treat with alpha-antagonists or 5 alpha reductase inhibitors
  - Surgery last option
- Acute testicular/scrotal pain
  - Consider torsion – if suspicious → surgery (no imaging). Absent cremasteric reflex very sensitive
  - Epididymitis and orchitis – may be due to chlamydia/gonorrhea
    - Treat with antimicrobials, acetaminophen, or NSAIDs
- Chronic prostatitis – α-blockers are effective treatment
- Hernias – palpated or visualized in inguinal canal
  - Surgical management

REFERENCES & SUGGESTED READINGS

1. U.S. Preventive Services Task Force. Screening for breast cancer: U.S. Preventive Services Task Force Recommendation Statement. *Ann Intern Med* 2009;151:716-726.

2. U.S. Preventive Services Task Force. *Screening for Colorectal Cancer: U.S. Preventive Services Task Force Recommendation Statement*. AHRQ Publication 08-05124-EF-3, October 2008. http://www.uspreventiveservicestaskforce.org/uspstf08/colocancer/colors.htm

3. *Screening for Cervical Cancer*, Topic Page. April 2012. U.S. Preventive Services Task Force. http://www.uspreventiveservicestaskforce.org/uspstf/uspscerv.htm

4. Centers for Disease Control and Prevention. Recommended adult immunization schedule—United States, 2012. MMWR 2012;61(4).

5. Fleisher LA, Beckman JA, Brown KA, Calkins H, Chaikof E, Fleischmann KE, Freeman WK, Froehlich JB, Kasper EK, Kersten JR, Riegel B, Robb JF. ACC/AHA 2007 guidelines on perioperative cardiovascular evaluation and care for noncardiac surgery: a report of the American College of Cardiology/American Heart Association Task Force on Practice Guidelines (Writing Committee to Revise the 2002 Guidelines on Perioperative Cardiovascular Evaluation for Noncardiac Surgery). *Circulation*. 2007;116:e418–e499.

6. McGlynn EA, et al. The quality of health care delivered to adults in the United States. *N Engl J Med*. 348:2635.

7. Snyder L, Leffler C; Ethics and Human Rights Committee; American College of Physicians. Ethics Manual: fifth edition. *Ann Intern Med*. 2005;142(7):560-582.

8. Qaseem A, Snow V, Shekelle P, et al; Clinical Efficacy Assessment Subcommittee of the American College of Physicians. Evidence-Based Interventions to Improve the Palliative Care of Pain, Dyspnea, and Depression at the End of Life: A Clinical Practice Guideline from the American College of Physicians. *Ann Intern Med*. 2008;148(2):141-146.

9. Keith M. Swetz, Arif H. Kamal, Deborah Cotton, Darren Taichman, Sankey Williams; Palliative Care. *Annals of Internal Medicine*. 2012 Feb;156(3):ITC2-1.

10. Irwin R, Madision JM. The Diagnosis and Treatment of Cough. *N Engl J Med*. 343:1715-1721.

11. Kapoor WN. Syncope. *N Engl J Med*. 343; 1856-1862.

12. Barbara Turner, Sankey Williams, Darren Taichman, Laurie Kopin, Charles Lowenstein; Dyslipidemia. *Annals of Internal Medicine*. 2010 Aug;153(3):ITC2-1.

13. Christine Laine, David R. Goldman, George A. Bray, Jennifer F. Wilson; Obesity. *Annals of Internal Medicine*. 2008 Oct;149(7):ITC4-1.

14. Daroff R. Dizziness and Vertigo. *Harrison's Principles of Internal Medicine*. 17th ed. Ed. Fauci A et al. New York: McGraw-Hill, 2008.

15. Fields HL and Martin JB. Pain: Pathophysiology and Management. *Harrison's Principles of Internal Medicine*. 17th ed. Ed. Fauci A et al. New York: McGraw-Hill, 2008.

NOTES

NOTES

2 **Pain Management**

Howard S. Smith, MD

Plinio P. Silva, MD, MPH

Contents

2.1 WHY PAIN MANAGEMENT

Though Pain Management is not expressly identified as a content area covered on the American Board of Internal Medicine (ABIM) certification exam, pain management can be found throughout many of the medical-content categories, including the 3% of the exam referred to as "Miscellaneous." Beyond exam study, we firmly believe that pain management knowledge is crucially important for healthcare providers in their day-to-day practice.

We have started the chapter with a section on over-the-counter (OTC), R_X, and alternative pain management. This section will help you understand drug-drug interactions at-a-glance, along with which OTC analgesics are safe and effective for certain pathologies, diseases, and symptoms. From there we will dive into an in-depth look at different pain areas.

2.2 INTRODUCTION

- The study of pain is defined by the International Association for the Study of Pain (IASP) as "an unpleasant sensory and emotional experience associated with actual or potential tissue damage, or described in terms of such damage"
- Acute pain is a physiologic response following a cascade of molecular events initiated by initial tissue injury
- Initially acute pain plays a protective role against further tissue damage, but can progress to a chronic disease if it persists despite apparent healing
- Acute and chronic pain are commonly encountered in clinical practice and present challenges to the internal medicine physician
- The 2011 Institute of Medicine (IOM) report, Relieving Pain in America: A Blueprint for Transforming Prevention, Care, Education, and Research:
    - Reported that pain affects as many as 100 million Americans and cost $635 billion annually
    - Called for a "cultural transformation" that would increase awareness and prevention; improve assessment and management; emphasize patient education; and address disparities in different patient subgroups

2.3 OTC, R_X, AND ALTERNATIVE PAIN MANAGEMENT

OTC Pain Medications

- Are used universally and benefit many patients
- Are generally safe and effective for short-term use when taken as directed
- Classes include:
    - Nonsteroidal anti-inflammatory drugs (NSAIDs):
        - Salicylates – an example is aspirin
        - Propionic acid derivatives – examples are ibuprofen, naproxen sodium, ketoprofen
    - Aminophenols – an example is acetaminophen
- Are used to treat mild to moderate pain
    - OTC pain medications treat pain that is commonly associated with many conditions including colds, flu, sore throat, headache, muscular aches, postoperative pain, arthritis, menstrual cramps, dental pain, and back pain

- Acetaminophen, an analgesic and antipyretic agent, does not have anti-inflammatory properties of NSAIDs. However, acetaminophen effectively treats mild to moderate pain without increasing the risk for gastrointestinal complications, such as gastric irritation, gastric erosions, bleeding, or ulcers when compared with NSAIDs
- As a medical professional, it is important to:
  - Know the precise amounts of all substances in an OTC formulation
  - Know the maximum daily dose of all agents contained in OTC formulations
  - Stay abreast of the latest evidence and dosing in order to give patient up-to-date advice and recommendations
  - Advise patients to communicate the exact quantity of OTC medications used
  - Counsel patients about the reason for use of the medication, frequency of administration, anticipated effect on symptoms, possible drug interactions, and potential adverse effects (especially severe ones)
  - Counsel patients to follow the labeled dosage and to not take more than the recommended labeled dose or the dose that is recommended by you, as this will help patients to prevent reaching toxic dose levels
  - Emphasize the importance of reading the package labeling sections
    - One of the FDA proposed changes requires that all OTC products containing NSAIDs or acetaminophen (including combination products) list these ingredients on the product's principal display panel and to also specify the potential for liver toxicity (in the case of acetaminophen) or GI complications (in the case of NSAIDs) when these products are taken with 3 or more alcoholic drinks daily
  - Monitor renal and liver function periodically
  - Educate parents and caregivers to keep OTC pain medications out of the reach of young children by storing these medicines in a high location that is out of the child's eye sight
  - Instruct the patient to avoid using more than 1 medicine that contains the same active ingredient at the same time
  - When recommending acetaminophen, inform patients of the following:
    - Advise patients to be mindful of alcoholic intake and discuss the use of alcohol while taking acetaminophen-containing medications, as liver damage may occur if the patient consumes more than the FDA's recommended amount of alcoholic consumption (3 or more drinks) each day while using acetaminophen. Again, patients should not exceed labeled dosing
    - Educate patients of the potential increased risk for bleeding if acetaminophen is taken with warfarin, a blood-thinning drug. Acetaminophen and warfarin combined may cause International Normalized Ratio (INR) elevation. Increased INR levels can be an indicator for early signs of internal bleeding
    - Instruct patients to ask you or a pharmacist when they are not sure whether a drug contains OTC pain relievers, such as acetaminophen. Also explain to the patient that severe liver damage may occur if the patient takes excessive amounts of acetaminophen, especially if the patient takes acetaminophen along with other drugs containing acetaminophen

- Further, educate patient regarding the existence of OTC medications that combine 2 or more active ingredients. Patients may not realize that the product contains 1 or more ingredient(s) that they are also taking in the form of another OTC or prescription medication, which may increase the risk of overdose. To reduce this problem, you may consider recommending a single-ingredient product whenever possible
  - When recommending NSAIDs, inform patients of the following:
    - Factors associated with the increased risk of NSAID-induced GI complications are older age, higher daily dosage, history of gastrointestinal or GI ulcer, history of GI hemorrhage, dyspepsia, NSAID intolerance, use of corticosteroids, use of anticoagulants, alcohol consumption, and poor general health
    - Individuals who have severe kidney or liver disease, hypertension, GI ulcers, or who take certain medications such as anticoagulants should not take OTC NSAIDs in order to reduce their risk for side effects
    - Advise patients with peptic ulcer disease to avoid taking NSAIDs for pain relief, as it increases the risk of gastrointestinal (GI) complications, ranging from mild dyspepsia to more severe problems such as gastrointestinal hemorrhage
    - NSAIDs with long-term use may cause renal injury. The use of aspirin, even low-dose aspirin, can affect renal function in the elderly. Therefore, NSAIDs should be used with caution in the elderly population because of the higher incidence of cardiovascular and GI disease, age-related decline in renal function and the likelihood of polypharmacy
    - Certain NSAIDs have drug-drug interactions with antihypertensive medications, which may result in elevated blood pressure and/or decrease in renal function. Therefore, advise patients with hypertension to avoid NSAIDs. Further, educate patients with hypertension regarding the use of acetaminophen for pain relief instead of NSAIDs while using antihypertensive medication. Acetaminophen does not affect blood pressure or have drug-drug interactions with antihypertensive medications
    - Ibuprofen and naproxen sodium may reduce the rate of renal clearance of lithium, increasing serum levels of lithium and an individual's risk for toxicity
    - Aspirin may potentiate hypoglycemic effects of sulfonylureas

Prescription Pain Medications (R$_X$)

- Widely used for treatment of moderate to severe acute and chronic pain
- Judicious prescription practices are important to decrease adverse effects of prescription pain medications
- Opioids used for the treatment of persistent non-cancer pain are of special importance given their abuse potential
- Inform patients of any side-effects and be aware of any OTC analgesic they are taking to avoid overdose
- The following practices are important prior to initiating chronic opioid therapy:
  - Informed consent
  - Opioid treatment agreement that includes a clause that opioids will be obtained from only 1 physician

- ° Goal directed therapy and periodic re-evaluation of treatment strategy are very important
- ° Evaluation of patients for abuse potential
  - Urine drug test
  - Psychological assessment
- ° Development of a strong doctor-patient relationship that will allow open communication

Complementary and Alternative Medicine (CAM)

- Emerging as potential adjuvant to conventional therapy in the treatment of chronic pain
- Acupuncture is the most widely used CAM modality
  - ° Acupuncture successfully employed for treatment of migraine and tension-type headaches, fibromyalgia, musculoskeletal pain, and pain during pregnancy
- Herbal medicine
  - ° Commonly used for the treatment of chronic pain
  - ° Treating physician must be aware of medicines to monitor for potential adverse effects and potential interactions with conventional medical therapies

Table 2.1: Common Drug-Drug Interactions Between OTC Pain Relievers and Prescription Drugs

OTC Pain Relievers	Prescription Drug	Common Drug-Drug Interactions
Acetaminophen and all NSAIDs	Warfarin	May increase the risk of bleeding
Acetaminophen	Isoniazid	Isoniazid prevents the metabolism of acetaminophen
All NSAIDs	Cyclosporine	NSAIDs reduce the renal clearance of cyclosporine, resulting in increased serum levels
All NSAIDs	Antihypertensives	NSAIDs may increase blood pressure and interact with antihypertensives. NSAIDs, such as aspirin, interact with antihypertensives (angiotensin-converting enzyme [ACE] inhibitors and β-blockers)
All NSAIDs	Methotrexate	NSAIDs may increase serum levels of methotrexate and lead to an increased risk of methotrexate toxicity
Ibuprofen and naproxen sodium	Lithium	Ibuprofen and naproxen sodium reduces the rate of renal clearance of lithium, increases serum levels of lithium, and may increase an individual's risk for toxicity
Aspirin	Sulfonylureas	Aspirin may potentiate hypoglycemic effects of sulfonylureas
Aspirin and other salicylates	Valproic acid	Aspirin and other salicylates reduce elimination of valproic acid, thus increasing the concentration of valproic acid in the blood. Due to the increased levels of valproic acid, valproic acid toxicity may occur

Adapted from Montauk SL, Rheinstein PH. Appropriate use of common OTC analgesics and cough and cold medications. Leawood, Kan.:American Academy of Family Physicians; 2002.

Table 2.2: OTC Pain Relievers With Certain Symptoms, Diseases, and Conditions*

Disease/Condition/Symptom	Preferred Analgesic	Therapeutic Note
Asthma	Acetaminophen	Use with caution: Aspirin, ibuprofen, naproxen sodium
Musculoskeletal (back, hip, elbow, shoulder, etc.) pain	Acetaminophen or ibuprofen	N/A
Bleeding disorders	Acetaminophen or non-aspirin salicylates	Use with caution: Aspirin, ibuprofen, naproxen sodium
Congestive heart failure	Acetaminophen	Use with caution: Effervescent aspirin tablets (with high sodium content), and non-salicylate NSAIDs
Dental pain	Ibuprofen. Alternative treatment includes acetaminophen	Use with caution: Aspirin or ibuprofen if extraction is planned
Dysmenorrhea	Ibuprofen, naproxen sodium, acetaminophen	N/A
Gout	Acetaminophen or non-salicylate NSAIDs	Use with caution: Salicylates
Headache	Acetaminophen, aspirin, or ibuprofen	N/A
Hepatic impairment	Acetaminophen	Use with caution: All NSAIDs
Hypertension	Acetaminophen	Use with caution: All NSAIDs
Lithium therapy	Acetaminophen or aspirin	Use with caution: Ibuprofen and naproxen sodium
Methotrexate therapy	Acetaminophen	Use with caution: All NSAIDs
Migraine	Ibuprofen or ASA. Alternative treatment includes acetaminophen	Avoid coated aspirin due to delayed onset
Acute sore throat pain (associated with upper respiratory tract infection), Pain (associated with the cold and flu)	Acetaminophen. Alternative treatment includes aspirin or ibuprofen	
Type 2 diabetes managed with 1st generation sulfonylureas	Acetaminophen or ibuprofen (however, patients with diabetes are at risk of renal dysfunction resulting from NSAID use)	Use with caution: Naproxen sodium, salicylates
Oral anticoagulant therapy	Acetaminophen or non-aspirin salicylates (patients taking anticoagulants who also take acetaminophen regularly or at higher doses should be monitored)	Use with caution: Aspirin, ibuprofen, naproxen sodium
Osteoarthritis or tendonitis	Acetaminophen or ibuprofen	
Peptic ulcer disease	Acetaminophen	Use caution with: All NSAIDs
Renal impairment	Acetaminophen	Use caution with: All NSAIDs
Rheumatoid arthritis	Acetaminophen, NSAIDs like ibuprofen and naproxen sodium	
Urticaria, Rash, Pruritic Rash	Acetaminophen	Salicylates

Adapted from: APhA. Self-Limited Pain Protocol Panel. APhA drug treatment protocols: self-care of self-limited pain. J Am Pharm Assoc. 1999;39:321-330.

Rowland, M. The pharmacist's role in pain relief. Pharmacy Post Clinical Report. June 2003.

*Labeled dosage should always be recommended unless otherwise suggested by the physician. Please refer to the Table on Drug-Drug Interactions of Common OTC Analgesics for additional information.

2.4 HEADACHE AND FACIAL PAIN

General Approach
- General history: Previous episodes, acuity, timing, severity, and medications
- Red flags: Very abrupt and severe (worst headache in patient's life), fever, focal neurological signs, and mental status changes such as cognitive dysfunction and diminished level of consciousness
- Physical exam (usually normal). Red flags: Neck stiffness, papilledema, or other focal deficits are concerning

Imaging
- Controversial and generally not helpful for diagnosis
- Indicated for patients with red flags on general history or physical exam
- Consider in the following settings:
  - Poor response or worsening in setting of appropriate therapy
  - New onset of headache in patients at extremes of age
  - Recent change in quality, severity, or timing of chronic headache
  - Association with exercise or other factors that would increase intracranial pressure (ICP)

Migraine
- High morbidity in general population
- Usually unilateral, gradual in onset, throbbing, lasts hours to days, and associated with significant impairment in function
- Aura (often visual), nausea, and vomiting are generally observed
- Photophobia and phonophobia are often present—pain is usually relieved by removal of these stimuli
- History alone is often enough to establish diagnosis

Acute Treatment for Migraine
- Trigger identification and avoidance
- Initial trial with nonsteroidal anti-inflammatory drugs (NSAIDs) or acetaminophen at labeled dosage
- If poor response, triptans and ergots are appropriate options
- If nausea and/or vomiting is severe enough to limit oral therapy, sumatriptan can be given subcutaneously or intranasally
- Early treatment may lead to improved outcomes

Prophylactic Treatment for Migraine
- Appropriate in patients with frequent attacks, long lasting attacks, and attacks associated with profound functional disability
- Improves control of migraine episodes
- Lowers incidence of analgesic rebound headache
- General classes used for prophylaxis:
  - Antihypertensives (β-blockers, ACE-I, calcium channel blockers)

- Antidepressants (amitriptyline, venlafaxine)
- Anticonvulsants (topiramate, valproate, gabapentin)
- Avoid opioids for prophylaxis given higher associated risk of chronic daily headache, dependence, and abuse potential

Tension-type Headache (TTH)
- Bilateral pressure of waxing and waning pattern and varying duration
- Degree of functional incapacitation is patient and episode dependent
- Associated with stress, anxiety, and depression

Acute Treatment for TTH
- Episodic TTH can be treated with analgesics agents:
  - Acetaminophen or NSAIDs like ibuprofen or naproxen sodium
  - Caffeine-containing combination agents can be used as second line therapy
- Severe TTH: Can be treated with intramuscular ketorolac
- Medications containing opioids, muscle relaxants, and triptans should be avoided

Prophylactic Treatment for TTH
- Mainstay of therapy is the tricyclic antidepressant (TCA) amitriptyline
- Mirtazapine and venlafaxine can be used as second line therapy
- Side effects are a major limiting factor

Patients with frequent episodic TTH are at high risk for developing medication overuse headache (MOH). Limit medication use and consider prophylactic therapy in the setting of frequent episodes.

Chronic Daily Headache
- Non-specific type of headache
  - Descriptive term that encompasses different subtypes of primary headaches
- Definition: Duration of 4 hours or longer, 15 days or more per month, and longer than 3 months without obvious organic cause
- 5 subtypes:
  1. Chronic migraine headache
  2. Chronic tension-type headache
  3. Medication overuse headache
  4. Hemicrania continua
  5. Daily persistent headache
- Diagnosis usually reached with full headache history and associated symptoms
- Treatment regimen dictated by specific headache type (e.g., botulinum toxin type A injections are Federal Drug Administration [FDA]-approved for chronic migraine headaches)

Trigeminal Autonomic Cephalalgias
- Multiple short lasting episodes—unilateral and severe
- Associated with autonomic symptoms (often ipsilateral)
  - Periorbital erythema and lacrimation
  - Rhinorrhea and nasal congestion
  - Facial diaphoresis and/or pallor

- ◦ Palpebral edema
- ◦ Horner's syndrome (rare)
- Very selective response to therapeutic approaches

Cluster Headache
Characteristics
- Deep periorbital or temporal pain with sudden progression
- Severe pain that is unilateral and bursting in quality
- Multiple cluster attacks a day lasting 15 minutes to 180 minutes
- Patients are usually restless and/or agitated
- May be accompanied by nausea, photophobia, and phonophobia
- More common in smokers and in men
- Alcohol intake may be a trigger

Acute Treatment for Cluster Headache
- First-line: 100% oxygen and subcutaneous sumatriptan. Intranasal route is also a viable option if subcutaneous (SQ) injection is contraindicated
- If no response or contraindication to sumatriptan—subcutaneous octreotide can be used

Prophylactic Treatment for Cluster Headache
- Start at onset of first episode to prevent/decrease further cluster episodes during same cluster period
- Active cluster period
  - ◦ <2 months, glucocorticoids alone is appropriate
  - ◦ >2 months, choose verapamil

Paroxysmal Hemicrania
Characteristics
- Sudden onset of severe periorbital or temporal pain
- Pain is sharp and throbbing
- Multiple attacks a day (up to 40) lasting 2 minutes to 30 minutes
- Possible nausea, photophobia, and phonophobia

Treatment for Paroxysmal Hemicrania
- Solely prophylactic as acute episodes are too short to be successfully treated
- Indomethacin is the mainstay of therapy

Short-lasting Unilateral Neuralgiform Headache (SUNCT) Attacks With Conjunctival Injection and Tearing
Characteristics of SUNCT
- Sudden onset of severe periorbital pain
- Pain is sharp and burning in quality
- Multiple attacks a day (up to 200) lasting from seconds to minutes
- May be triggered by cutaneous stimulation

Acute Treatment of SUNCT
- Intravenous lidocaine

Prophylactic Treatment of SUNCT
- Lamotrigine, topiramate, or gabapentin

Trigeminal Neuralgia (TN)

- 2 etiology categories
  - 1. Classic: Idiopathic or associated with vascular compression
    - Diagnostic criteria
      - Paroxysmal attacks of pain lasting from less than a second up to 2 minutes
      - Affects 1 or more divisions of Trigeminal (V) nerve
      - At least 1 of the following:
        - Pain is stabbing, sharp, severe, and superficial
        - Triggered by focal stimulation or other trigger factors
      - Attacks are similar or same in the individual patient (stereotyped) followed by refractory period
      - No obvious clinical neurologic deficit
      - Not caused by another disorder
  - 2. Secondary: Caused by diagnosed structural lesion that is not related to the vasculature
    - Pain essentially indistinguishable from Classic TN
    - Cause is a structural lesion that is not associated with vascular compression
    - No refractory period following attack
    - May be associated with sensory impairment of affected region (trigeminal branch)
- Utility of imaging is controversial, but may be useful in distinguishing Classic from Secondary TN

Treatment of TN

- Medical therapy is first-line treatment
  - Classic TN: Carbamazepine, oxcarbazepine, baclofen
- Surgical therapy is reserved to TN that is refractory to medical therapy
  - Microvascular decompression
  - Nerve ablation
    - Rhizotomy
    - Gamma knife radiosurgery
    - Peripheral neurectomy and nerve block

Headache Secondary to Changes in Intracranial Pressure or Volume

Idiopathic Intracranial Hypertension (Pseudotumor Cerebri)

- Highest incidence seen in overweight/obese women of childbearing age
- Headache
  - The most common symptom
  - Pain is generally described as unilateral, severe, and throbbing
  - Often confused with other diagnosis: Migraines, TTH, MOH
- Other associated signs and symptoms: Papilledema, vision loss (especially visual field loss that can then be followed by visual acuity loss), diplopia, pulse synchronous tinnitus, retrobulbar pain, cranial nerve (CN) palsy (especially the abducens nerve – CN VI)
- Symptoms are thought to be secondary to increase in ICP
- Initial evaluation must rule out other causes of increased ICP (mass lesion, obstruction of cerebrospinal fluid (CSF) outflow, increased CSF production)
- Treatment: Symptom management and prevention of vision loss

Thunderclap Headache (TCH)

- Severe, sudden headache ("In a clap of thunder")

- Requires urgent evaluation to rule out secondary cause, especially subarachnoid hemorrhage

Etiologies of Secondary Thunderclap Headache
1. Subarachnoid hemorrhage
2. Unruptured intracranial aneurysm (sentinel headache)
3. Cerebral venous thrombosis
4. Cervical artery dissection
5. Spontaneous intracranial hypotension
6. Pituitary apoplexy
7. Retroclival hematoma
8. Ischemic stroke
9. Acute hypertensive crisis
10. Colloid cyst of the third ventricle
11. Infection (encephalitis, meningitis)
12. Cerebral vasoconstrictions

If secondary cause ruled out, then a diagnosis of primary thunderclap headache can be considered.

Primary Thunderclap Headache Diagnostic Criteria
- Pain is severe, sudden in onset reaching maximum intensity in less than a minute
- Pain lasts from 1 hour to 10 days
- May recur during the 1st week, but not over the following weeks or months
- Not secondary to any other disorder

In addition to standard clinical evaluation, studies used to help elucidate the etiology of TCH include: Computerized axial tomography (CT) scan, lumbar puncture, magnetic resonance imaging (MRI), magnetic resonance angiography (MRA), and angiography.

2.5 CHRONIC MUSCULOSKELETAL PAIN AND OTHER COMMON CHRONIC PAIN CAUSES

Low Back Pain
- 1 of the most common reasons for outpatient clinic visits
- Often seen in patients ages 35 to 55
- Low back pain is classified as:
  ◦ Acute: 2 to 4 weeks
  ◦ Subacute: <12 weeks
  ◦ Chronic: >12 weeks
- Risk factors: Psychological or physical stress, heavy lifting, smoking, obesity, and psychiatric illness (depression and anxiety)
- History and physical examination are very important with special focus to rule out systemic disease as a primary cause
- Red flags associated with systemic disease: Older age, cancer history, weight loss, pain >30 days, or poor response to therapy

- Imaging is usually not helpful early in course of disease, as most episodes are self-resolving
  - Imaging is indicated if pain persists for >4 to 6 weeks
    - Plain film of spine should be done first, followed by CT/MRI if necessary
  - CT/MRI helpful if pain persists for >12 weeks or if there is a high suspicion of systemic disease (especially cancer and red flags listed)

Treatment of Low Back Pain

Acute Low Back Pain
- Usually has an excellent prognosis
- Avoid bed rest
- Treatment: Reasonable first-line analgesic choice is acetaminophen to help treat symptoms and improve mobility. NSAIDs may also be considered, but there is an associated higher incidence of side effects (see OTC, R_x, and Alternative Pain Management). Muscle relaxants such as cyclobenzaprine can also be considered
- If pain persists, initial therapy with opioids can be helpful; however, short course of scheduled around the clock therapy is preferred over an as-needed (PRN) basis

Subacute and Chronic Low Back Pain
- Evaluate for cause based on history and clinical assessment as outlined above
- Avoid bed rest
- Treatment with NSAIDs or acetaminophen during exacerbation
- Limit opioids to short courses of scheduled therapy and to patients with low abuse potential
- Assess and treat exacerbating factors and co-morbid conditions: Psychosocial stress, depression, and anxiety
- A trial of tricyclic antidepressants may be of benefit even for those not suffering with depression
- Exercise has been shown to be beneficial, including yoga, aerobic, and physical therapy
- Surgery generally not recommended. Early benefits usually seen but these usually do not persist

Neck Pain
- Spontaneous or traumatic in origin
- Usually secondary to cervical spine disease or soft tissue injury:
  - Myofascial pain
  - Cervical radiculopathy with or without spinal stenosis
  - Axial pain or facet joint arthrosis
- Red flags: Fever, cancer history (with or without metastasis), and rapid progression of symptoms
- Rule out neurologic compromise by physical examination
- Multifaceted therapy is best approach:
  - Pharmacotherapy: Acetaminophen or NSAIDs are first-line treatments
    - Muscle relaxant can be added if spasms are evident
  - Physical therapy with postural correction and rest
  - Elimination of ongoing stress or inciting factors
- If poor response to above therapy and unclear diagnosis, more thorough evaluation for neuropathic component of pain is necessary
  - Burning pain with weakness, numbness, and loss of reflexes
  - Can be treated with antidepressants

- Moderate, chronic, and refractory pain can be treated with trigger point injections, surgery, and opioids

Shoulder Pain

- Common complaint that affects majority of adults at some point in life
- Deep, ache-like pain on lateral arm at point of deltoid insertion (referred pain)
- Also associated with difficulty abducting arm above level of the head, pain with pressure on shoulder area (sleeping on affected side), and reaching towards their back
- Important to evaluate for history of trauma, overuse, or other inciting factor
- All patients should be evaluated with a plain film radiograph
- Traumatic injury should be treated with reduction (closed or open) and immobilization
- Specific therapy depends on diagnosis
- Non-traumatic injury can be treated with:
    - Rest and NSAIDs or acetaminophen for symptomatic relief
    - Gentle exercises followed by strengthening exercises and possible physical therapy

Differential Diagnosis

- Fracture
- Dislocation
- Impingement
- Acromioclavicular arthritis
- Biceps tendinitis
- Rotator cuff tear
- Instability
- Superior labrum anterior posterior lesion
- Frozen shoulder
- Cervical disk

Elbow Pain

- Presentation depends on etiology and final diagnosis
- Most common diagnosis and associated presentations
    - Epicondylitis (lateral vs. medial)
        - Local tenderness at muscle origin and/or tendon
        - Pain worse in morning and associated with tearing sensation
        - Secondary to avascular necrosis of common extensor or flexor tendon
        - Treatment: Rest, ice, splinting, NSAIDs or acetaminophen, possible steroid injection, possible surgery
    - Ulnar neuropathy
        - Elbow pain and tenderness that is medially located (where ulnar nerve courses medial epicondyle)
        - Associated with hypoesthesia in the ulnar nerve distribution (medial half of 4th digit and the 5th digit), can progress to hand weakness secondary to intrinsic muscle atrophy
        - Treatment: Rest, therapy, gliding of ulnar nerve
    - Ulnar nerve subluxation
        - Snapping sensation with elbow flexion and extension
        - Paresthesias, especially shock like sensation, in ulnar distribution
        - Treatment: Rest, flexion avoidance, and possible surgery if it persists

- Radial nerve/peripheral interosseous nerve compression
  - Deep, ache like pain, distributed over extensor surface of forearm
  - Treatment: Rest, therapy, gliding of radial nerve, and surgical decompression may be needed
- Elbow instability
  - Traumatic dislocation or repetitive injury (exercise)
  - Treatment: Physical therapy
- Fracture
  - Associated with acute trauma
  - Treatment: Reduction and immobilization, possibly open reduction and internal fixation (ORIF)
- Synovitis
  - Associated with elbow swelling and painful flexion/extension
  - Treatment: Rest, ice, splinting, NSAID therapy, steroid injection, possible surgery
- Arthritis
  - Trauma or history of inflammation (rheumatoid arthritis)
  - Treatment: Rest, ice, splinting, acetaminophen as first-line therapy before trying NSAIDs, possible steroid injection, possible surgery
- Olecranon bursitis
  - Inflammation of olecranon bursa
  - Localized swelling on posterior forearm at elbow
  - Treatment: Usually self-limiting so observation is warranted, antibiotics are indicated if cellulitis is present, incision and drainage (I&D) with bursectomy if no improvement or systemic symptoms are seen

Wrist and Hand Pain

Carpal Tunnel Syndrome
- Common cause of upper extremity neuropathy
- Pain and/or symptoms result from compression of median nerve
- Presents with hand paresthesia and/or hypoesthesia in the distribution of median nerve
  - Palmar surface – 1st digit to lateral half of 4th digit
  - Dorsal surface – 2nd digit to 4th digit distal to the distal interphalangeal joints (DIP)
- Can eventually progress to thenar muscles weakness and atrophy
- Treatment
  - Start conservatively with wrist splinting, NSAIDs or acetaminophen, diuretics, and possible steroid injection
  - If conservative treatment fails then surgical release of transverse carpal ligament can be performed

Ulnar Tunnel Syndrome
- Caused by compression of ulnar nerve in Guyon's canal (fascial band between pisiform and hamate)
- Presents with paresthesia and hypoesthesia in 5th digit and medial half of 4th digit
- Can be seen in long distance cyclers, prolonged use of screwdrivers and pliers, golfers, and racquet sports players
- Treatment: Rest, avoiding inciting factors, splinting, NSAIDs, steroid injections, occupational therapy, and ultimately surgery if conservative treatment fails

Cubital Tunnel Syndrome
- Most common site of ulnar nerve compression
- Injury can develop after prolonged elbow flexion, compression secondary to osteoarthritis or inappropriate growth after elbow fracture
- Patients usually present with medial elbow pain and paresthesia radiating to the 4th and 5th digits
- Can eventually progress to intrinsic hand weakness (grip strength)
- Treatment: Sling with immobilization to avoid elbow flexion, decreasing activities that involve elbow flexion, and possible treatment with NSAIDs or acetaminophen

Referred Pain
- Hand pain can be a presentation of myocardial infarction or stable/unstable angina as referred pain, especially when associated with activity
- Cervical disk disease
  - Usually presents with pain radiating from cervical area to hand
  - Pain path usually follows distribution of nerve root being compressed

Hip Pain

Trochanteric Bursitis
- Inflammation of trochanteric bursa
- Presents as lateral pain that is worsened by pressure/palpation
- Treatment: Localized physical therapy, NSAIDs, and rest

Hip Arthritis
- Generally presents as pain radiating to groin that is worsened by movement of hip joint and relieved by rest
- Eventually leads to decreased range of motion
- Can be caused by many factors, such as osteoarthritis, osteonecrosis, trauma, sepsis, and rheumatoid arthritis
- Treatment
  - Initially conservative with rest, physical therapy, acetaminophen or NSAIDs, and physical support (i.e., cane in opposite hand)
  - If obesity is present, weight loss can significantly improve pain
  - Surgical treatment with total joint replacement may eventually become necessary if pain is refractory to conservative measures

Avascular Necrosis (AVN)
- Etiology is generally unknown
- Associated with alcohol intake, steroid use, trauma, and sickle cell disease (S or SC)
- Presents as groin pain and/or a limp
- Treatment largely surgical, although initially analgesics and physical support can be helpful

Occult Hip Fracture
- Usually secondary to osteoporosis
- More common in women
- Generally associated with previous trauma (even if minor)
- Presents as hip/groin pain and inability to bear weight on affected side
- Treatment is surgical stabilization of femoral head and treatment of osteoporosis to decrease likelihood of future fractures

Malignancy
- Presents as constant pain generally not associated with activity
- Can be site of primary malignancy or metastasis (especially in patients with a history of cancer)
- Treatment: Surgical intervention may decrease likelihood of future fractures

Infection
- Presents with constant joint pain associated with decrease in movement of joint, inability to bear weight, and generally worse at night
- Fevers and history of bacteremia are helpful in making diagnosis
- Generally presents with elevated white blood cells (WBC), c-reactive protein (CRP), and erythrocyte sedimentation rate (ESR)
- Aspiration of joint effusion can aid greatly in diagnosis with analysis of aspirate
- Treatment: Intravenous (IV) antibiotics and pain relief

Knee Pain

Patellofemoral Syndrome
- Presents as anterior knee pain exacerbated by prolonged sitting
- Secondary to trauma, overuse or poor alignment of patella and femur resulting in repetitive irritation
- Treatment
    - Analgesic medication, commonly restricted to acetaminophen or aspirin, for 3 to 4 weeks, followed by a taper
    - For refractory pain, corticosteroid injections and surgery are options

Pes Anserine Bursitis
- Presents as anteromedial knee pain
- Usually caused by an abnormal gait or trauma resulting in inflammation of the bursa between the pes anserine tendons and the medial collateral ligament (MCL)
- Treatment
    - Address abnormal gait, ice, and avoidance of knee flexion. NSAIDs can be used for pain but low vasculature in this region may prevent adequate therapeutic effect
    - If pain persists for more than 6 to 8 weeks, local anesthetic and methylprednisolone injections are used second as second-line

Prepatellar Bursitis
- Presents with anterior knee pain and a swollen knee
- Often caused by trauma or after prolonged and frequent pressure, such as kneeling
- Can also be caused by urate crystal accumulation
- Knee range of motion is generally preserved
- Aspiration should be done to rule out infectious or crystal induced arthropathy etiology and as a therapeutic measure
- Treatment
    - Aspiration to reduce pressure and pain, compression dressing, ice, NSAIDs, and avoidance of knee flexion
    - 40% will require corticosteroid injection once infection and gout are ruled out
    - 5% will go on to develop chronic bursitis and may require a bursectomy

Iliotibial Band Tendinitis
- Presents as lateral knee pain

- Common sport-associated injury (e.g., running, cycling)
- Caused by repetitive friction of a tight iliotibial band with the lateral femoral condyle
- Treatment: Ice, rest, NSAIDs or acetaminophen, and progressive stretching of iliotibial band

Osteoarthritis
- Presents as knee pain that is worsened by activity and relieved by rest, and morning stiffness that improves with activity
- An effusion is often present
- Predisposing factors: Family history, obesity, genu valgum, genu varum, previous knee trauma, or injury to meniscus
- Treatment
    - Rest, ice, elevation, avoiding repetitive impact and physical therapy aiming at strengthening the quadriceps muscle. In addition, glucosamine sulfate and acetaminophen or NSAID course with taper
    - If pain is refractory to above treatment, a second NSAID course with a different NSAID can be attempted along with local injection of corticosteroid and local anesthetic
    - Surgical reconstruction of the knee joint is indicated when pain is refractory to conservative treatment, severe disability, cartilage destruction reaches 80 to 90% or the patient develops angulation of lower extremity
- Popliteal Cyst (Baker's Cyst)
    - Presents with posterior knee pain associated with popliteal fossa distention and hypoesthesia
    - Over time, recurrent effusions can result in a protrusion of the posterior capsule into the posterior fossa and subsequent cyst formation
    - Treatment targeted towards identifying and treating source of effusion
    - Surgical therapy is necessary if cyst persists or venous compression is identified

Remember: Acute knee pain secondary to trauma can be a result of injuries to anterior cruciate ligament (ACL), posterior cruciate ligament (PCL), medial collateral ligament (MCL), lateral collateral ligament (LCL), or meniscus. In addition, the differential of acute knee pain includes septic arthritis, gout and pseudogout.

Ankle and Foot Pain

Tarsal Tunnel Syndrome
- Caused by entrapment of posterior tibial nerve or its branches (medial calcaneal nerve, medial plantar nerve, lateral plantar nerve, and first branch of lateral plantar nerve)
- Nerve compression can occur before or after terminal branch division
- Usually presents with medial mid foot pain
- Roughly half of patients may have a positive Tinel's sign
- Compression of the lateral plantar nerve occurs most often (e.g., Jogger's foot) and causes stabbing pain in the medial sole when walking or running
- Treatment
    - Conservative: NSAIDs, icing, massage, shoe modification, steroid injections
    - Surgical release

Arthritis
- Inflammatory or osteoarthritis
- Rheumatoid arthritis affecting the foot and ankle can be seen in up to 90% of cases
- Gout and pseudogout are commonly seen involving the foot
  - Treatment may include: NSAIDs or acetaminophen, colchicines, steroid injection
- Osteoarthritis of foot and ankle usually involves the first MTP joint and naviculocuneiform, intercuneiform, and metatarsocuneiform joints
  - Treatment: NSAIDs or acetaminophen and shoe modification

Plantar Fasciitis
- Inflammation of foot plantar fascia
- Chronic plantar fasciitis is usually characterized by marked collagen degeneration
- Pain and tenderness may be maximal over the origin of the plantar fascia on the medial calcaneal tuberosity and along the fascia 1 cm to 2 cm distal to the origin
- Associated with obesity, foot deformities, and middle age
- Typically presents with pain at the distal portion of the heel pad (calcaneus) that is worse in the morning or when standing after rest
- Treatment modalities vary and include: Ice, rest, casting, NSAIDs or acetaminophen, possible steroid injections, physical therapy, and orthotics
- Most cases resolve after a period of conservative treatment

Other Heel and Foot Pain
- Morton's metatarsalgia (Morton's neuroma)
  - Lancinating, shock-like pain between the 3rd and 4th toes upon mechanical stress
- Calcaneal stress fracture
  - Progressively worsening heel pain
  - Usually follows increase in activity level or change to a harder walking and/or exercise surface
- Heel pad syndrome (fat pad atrophy)
  - Deep, bruise like pain in the mid heel area usually most intense over central portion of heel fat pad
  - Without medial calcaneal tuberosity and plantar fascia tenderness
- Achilles tendinopathy
  - Posterior heel pain
- Sinus tarsi syndrome
  - Anterolateral ankle pain and/or lateral midfoot heel pain
  - Usually secondary to excessive motions of the subtalar joint or trauma
  - Results in subtalar joint synovitis and infiltration of fibrotic tissue into the sinus tarsi space (anterior to lateral malleolus)
- Calcaneal periostitis
  - Pain and tenderness over calcaneus
- Haglund deformity related pain
  - A prominence of the calcaneus that may cause bursa inflammation between the calcaneus and Achilles tendon

2.6 OTHER TYPES OF COMMON CHRONIC PAIN

Chronic Functional Abdominal Pain

- Defined as continuous or almost continuous pain without evidence of organic disease that has been present for 6 months, and interferes with daily functions
- The cause of chronic functional abdominal pain is poorly understood but may be due to the persistence of nerve sensitization after an initial event such as surgery or inflammation
- Chronic functional abdominal pain is generally a diagnosis of exclusion. A broad differential must first be ruled out
- The psychosocial aspect of chronic functional abdominal pain is also very important to consider
- Treatment varies but generally includes multimodal therapeutic approaches with physical, occupational, behavioral therapies, and medications
- Avoid use of opioids and barbiturates

Fibromyalgia Syndrome

- Pain-amplification syndrome in highly sensitive patients
  - Both sensory abnormalities and psychosocial exacerbating factors have been described
- A widespread chronic pain that is present for greater than 3 months and upon examination, elicits painful response at 10 or more of the 18 tender points: Occiput area, upper back/neck, upper chest, elbows hips, and knees
- Patients present with widespread pain, chronic fatigue and other debilitating conditions such as stress, anxiety, depression, irritable bowel syndrome, or headaches
- Diagnosis must only be made after significant work-up for other causes of pain
- Treatment
  - Medication based treatment
    - Tricyclic antidepressants
    - Selective serotonin reuptake inhibitors (SSRIs) and serotonin-norepinephrine reuptake inhibitors (SNRIs)
    - Lidocaine trigger point injection
    - Pregabalin and gabapentin
  - Non medication treatment
    - Low to moderate intensity exercise has been shown to improve physical symptoms and functional capacity
    - Extensive patient education is also beneficial

2.7 ACUTE AND CHRONIC PAIN IN DIFFERENT PATIENT POPULATIONS

Women and Pain

- Women may have higher prevalence of chronic pain conditions
- Evidence suggests that the pathophysiology and experience of chronic pain in women is different than chronic pain in men. This is thought to be secondary to the expression of different pain receptors
- Spinal cord Mu opioid receptor and Kappa opioid receptor heterodimers may represent unique targets for providing analgesia in women

- Rates of oral and or facial pain, migraines, and fibromyalgia are higher in women when compared to rates of the same conditions in men
- Pathologies specific to women
  - Menstrual migraines
  - Chronic pelvic pain
- OTC treatments
  - NSAIDs for short-term treatment reduce swelling and relieve pain
  - Non-opioid analgesic acetaminophen reduces fever, relieves pain due to headaches, back pain, sore muscles, and joint pain; can be used in combination with opioid medications
- Pregnancy and OTC analgesics
  - Acetaminophen: 1st/2nd/3rd trimesters - Category B
  - Non-salicylate NSAIDs: 1st and/or 2nd trimester - Category B; 3rd trimester – Category D
  - Aspirin should generally be avoided
  - Analgesics should be used in the smallest, most effective dose for pain relief
- Breastfeeding
  - Acetaminophen and non-salicylate NSAIDs are considered safe
  - Salicylates can be excreted in human milk
  - The use of high doses of aspirin can produce effects in the nursing infant

Ethnic Differences
- Significant disparities exist on the treatment of pain in minority groups
- Minority groups are less likely to be prescribed opioid therapy for severe pain
  - Minority patients are at risk for under-treatment of acute pain across life span and treatment settings
- They receive less analgesic therapy in general
- Pain management and assessment have also been found to be less than adequate for minority groups in emergency department settings
- Different ethnic groups may have slightly different expression of drug metabolizers leading to higher or lower drug levels than those seen in other patients
  - This is particularly important with codeine, as a patient who has decreased expression of the CYP2D6 will not be able to convert codeine (pro-drug) to morphine, its active metabolite. Therefore these patients will not receive appropriate therapeutic benefit

Pain in the Pediatric Patient
- Assessment of pain, especially chronic pain, in the pediatric patients is challenging
- Many tools are available to facilitate evaluation
- In older children, self-report can also be reliably used
- Treatment
  - Nonpharmacologic: Psychosocial, cognitive behavioral therapy, parental education, and support
  - Pharmacologic
    - Organ development, different body composition and plasma protein levels must be taken into consideration (especially in neonates) for drug metabolism, clearance, and plasma concentrations

- Acetaminophen
  - Common use in pediatrics because of excellent safety profile and few side effects, if taken at labeled dosage
  - Often combined with opioids for the treatment of moderate/severe pain
  - Weight dosing is extremely important to avoid toxicity
- NSAIDs
  - Pharmacology is similar in children and adults
  - Children have lower incidence of renal and gastrointestinal (GI) associated adverse effects
  - Ibuprofen is commonly used for treatment of mild/moderate pain, and ketorolac is often used for treatment of acute pain
- Opioids
  - Dosing is dependent on the child's age as plasma clearance and drug metabolism vary accordingly
  - Children are at greater risk for developing respiratory distress secondary to opioids administration and should always be monitored

Geriatrics and Chronic Pain

- Patient population frequently affected by chronic pain
- Pharmacokinetic and pharmacodynamic changes with age are important to consider
  - Acetaminophen and NSAIDs
    - No adjustment in labeled dosage is necessary for older patients who take acetaminophen for mild to moderate musculoskeletal pain
    - NSAIDs are associated with GI ulcers, bleeding, and gastrointestinal perforation
    - Acetaminophen is a better choice for relief of pain from osteoarthritis because of decreased risk of gastrointestinal problems
    - The effects of NSAIDs on prostaglandin synthesis can significantly interfere with the effects of many different types of antihypertensive medications that the geriatric patient uses including: Diuretics, β-blockers, ACE inhibitors, vasodilators, central alpha-agonists and peripheral alpha-antagonists
- Elderly patients show different patterns of drug distribution due to different body composition, lower muscle mass, and total body water but increased fat mass
- Elderly may be more sensitive to higher doses of opioids and exercising caution with slow increase in doses is safer

Alcohol Use and OTC Analgesics

- Chronic heavy alcohol abusers may be at increased risk of liver toxicity from excessive acetaminophen use. Therefore, healthcare professionals should inform their patients who regularly consume large amounts of alcohol not to exceed recommended doses of acetaminophen
- The concurrent use of alcohol and NSAIDs has been associated with an increased risk of GI bleeding and increases an individual's risk ratio for developing gastrointestinal complications than alcohol abuse or NSAID use alone

- Approximately 15% of patients treated with NSAIDs have borderline elevations of serum transaminases, LDH, and alkaline phosphatase. NSAIDs are highly protein-bound and some are extensively metabolized by the liver. Metabolic activity and/or plasma protein binding may be altered in patients with hepatic impairment, which may result in a dosage reduction for some patients
- The combination of acetaminophen and alcohol, especially moderate to heavy alcohol use, may result in a significant risk of hepatotoxicity. However, hepatotoxicity with acetaminophen occurs almost exclusively in the setting of massive overdose. Therefore, advise patient to strictly adhere to dosing as indicated on the medication label
- Patients should be counseled about the risks of combining alcohol and OTC pain relievers and be encouraged to not exceed the recommended label daily dose of these medications
- When communicating with patients about the use of OTC pain medications and discussing responsible dosing, especially if alcohol use is involved, it is important for you to:
  - Address with patients the responsible use of products containing acetaminophen and NSAIDs
  - Inform patients about the potential risks of the NSAIDs and acetaminophen
  - Educate patients to always read package labeling and follow the label carefully
    - Emphasize the importance of reading the package labeling sections labeled "Warnings and Directions." One of the FDA proposed changes requires that all OTC products containing NSAIDs or acetaminophen (including combination products) to list these ingredients on the product's principal display panel and to also specify the potential for liver toxicity (in the case of acetaminophen) or GI complications (in the case of NSAIDs) when these products are taken with 3 or more alcoholic drinks daily
  - Counsel patients to follow the labeled dosage and to not take more than the recommended labeled dose or the dose that is recommended by you, as this will help patients to prevent reaching toxic dose levels
  - Stay current on OTC usage patterns, trends, proper storage, and risks with improper use of OTC drugs because of the high occurrence of OTC medication use
  - Instruct patients to ask you or a pharmacist when they are not sure whether a drug contains acetaminophen. Inform patients that severe liver damage may occur if taken with other drugs containing acetaminophen

REFERENCES & SUGGESTED READING

1. Lipton RB et al. Classification of Primary Headaches. *Neurology*. 2004;63:427.

2. Goadsby PJ. To Scan or Not to Scan. *BMJ*. 2004;329:469.

3. Silberstein SD, Rosenberg J. Multispecialty Consensus on Diagnosis and Treatment of Headache. *Neurology*. 2000;54:1553.

4. Derry S, et al. Paracetamol (Acetaminophen) With or Without Antiemetic for Acute Migraine Headaches in Adults. *Cochrane Database Syst Rev*. 2010; CD008040.

5. Lipton RB, et al. Efficacy and Safety of Acetaminophen in the Treatment of Migraine: Results of a Randomized, Double-blind, Placebo-controlled, Population-based Study. *Arch Intern Med*. 2000;160:3486.

6. Lipton RB et al. Efficacy and Safety of Acetaminophen, Aspirin, and Caffeine in Alleviating Migraine Headache Pain: Three Double-blind, Randomized, Placebo-controlled trials. *Arch Neurol*. 1998;55: 210.

7. Silberstein SD. Practice Parameter: Evidence-based Guidelines for Migraine Headache (An Evidence-based Review): Report of the Quality Standards Subcommittee of the American Academy of Neurology. *Neurology*. 2000;55:754.

8. Linde K, et al. Acupuncture for Migraine Prophylaxis. *Cochrane Database Syst Review*. 2009;CD001218.

9. Headache subcommittee of the International Headache Society. The International Classification of Headache Disorders: 2nd edition. *Cephalalgia*. 2004;24:9.

10. May A, et al. EFNS Guidelines on the Treatment of Cluster Headache and Other Trigeminal-autonomic Cephalalgias. *Eur J Neurology*. 2006;13:1066.

11. Bendtsen L, et al. EFNS Guideline on the Treatment of Tension-type Headache. *Curr Pain Headache*. 2003;7:466.

12. Dodick DW, et al. Clinical Practice. Chronic Daily Headache. *NEJM*. 2006;354:158.

13. Friedman DI, et al. Diagnostic Criteria for Idiopathic Intracranial Hypertension. *Neurology*. 2002;59:1492.

14. Reitsma M, et al. The epidemiology of chronic pain in Canadian men and women between 1994 and 2007: Longitudinal Results of the National Population Health Survey. *Pain Res Manag*. 2012;17:166.

15. Smith, Howard. Current Therapy in Pain. Philadelphia, Pa: Saunders Elsevier; 2009.

16. Smith, Howard. Opioid Therapy. In:The 21st Century. New York, NY: Oxford University Press; 2008.

17. Benzon, Honorio, et al. Essentials of Pain Medicine. Philadelphia, Pa: Saunders Elsevier; 2011.

18. Young SS. Appropriate use of common OTC analgesics and cough and cold medications. Leawood, Ks: American Academy of Family Physicians; 2002.

19. Pharmacy Links. The pharmacist's role in pain relief. Pharmacy Post Clinical Report. Available at: http://www.pharmacylinksonline.com/images/06_PPO_17_21.pdf. Accessed September 16, 2012.

20. Recommendations for the medical management of osteoarthritis of the hip and knee: 2000 update. American College of Rheumatology Subcommittee on Osteoarthritis Guidelines. *Arthritis Rheum*. 2000;43(9):1905-1915.

21. U.S. Department of Health and Human Services. Managing Osteoarthritis: Helping the Elderly Maintain Function and Mobility. Available at: http://www.ahrq.gov/research/osteoria/osteoria.htm. Accessed September 16, 2012.

22. Anderson KO, Green CR, Payne R. Racial and Ethnic Disparities in Pain: Causes and Consequences of Unequal Care. *The Journal of Pain*. 2009; 10(12):1187-1204.

23. WebMD. Chronic Pain: OTC or Prescription Medicine? Available at: http://www.webmd.com/pain-management/features/when-to-call--doctor?print=true. Accessed September 16, 2012.

24. WebMD. Plantar Fasciitis. Available at: http://www.webmd.com/a-to-z-guides/plantar-fasciitis-when-to-call-a-doctor?print=true. Accessed September 16, 2012.

25. Hudes K. Conservative management of a case of tarsal tunnel syndrome. *J Can Chiropr Assoc*. 2010; 54(2):100-106.

26. Emedicine-Medscape. Iliotibial Band Friction Syndrome Treatment and Management. Available at: http://emedicine.medscape.com/article/1250716-treatment. Accessed September 17, 2012.

27. Emedicine-Medscape. Prepatellar Bursitis Medication. Available at: http://emedicine.medscape.com/article/309014-medication. Accessed September 17, 2012.

28. Emedicine-Medscape. Pes Anserine Bursitis Treatment and Management. Available at: http://emedicine.medscape.com/article90412-treatment. Accessed September 17, 2012.

29. Nursing Times. Swift A. Osteoarthritis 2: pain management and treatment strategies. Available at: http://www.nursingtimes.net/osteoarthritis-2-pain-management-and-treatment-strategies/50. Accessed September 16, 2012.

30. Merck Manual. Nerve compression Syndromes. Available at: http://www.merckmanuals.com/professional/print/musculoskeletal_and_connective_tissue. Accessed September 17, 2012.

31. Emedicine-Medscape. Trochanteric Bursitis Medication. Available at: http://emedicine.medscape.com/article/87788-medication. Accessed September 17, 2012.

32. American Academy of Orthopaedic Surgeries. Ulnar Tunnel Syndrome of the Wrist. Available at: http://orthoinfo.aaos.org/topic.cfm?topic=a00025. Accessed September 16, 2012.

33. American College of Rheumatology. Carpal Tunnel Syndrome. Available at: http://www.rheumatology.org/pracice/clinical/patients/diseases_and_conditions/carpaltunnel. Accessed September 16, 2012.

34. Emedicine-Medscape. Avascular Necrosis Treatment and Management. Available at: http://emedicine.medscape.com/article/333364-treatment. Accessed September 16, 2012.

35. Brandt KD, Mazzuca SA, Buckwalter KA. Acetaminophen, like conventional NSAIDs, may reduce synovitis in osteoarthritic knees. *Rheumatology*. 2006;45(11):1389-1394.

36. Emedicine-Medscape. Patellofemoral Syndrome Medication. Available at: http://emedicine.medscape.com/article/308471-medication. Accessed September 16, 2012.

37. Feleus A, Bierma-Zeinstra S, Miedema H, Verhaar J, Koes B. Management in non-traumatic arm, neck and shoulder complaints: differences between diagnostic groups. *Eur Spine J*. 2008;17(9):1218-1229.

NOTES

NOTES

3 Otorhinolaryngology: Ear, Nose, & Throat

Sarah Boutwell, MD

Dary Costa, MD

Jastin Antisdel, MD

Contents

3.1 EVALUATION OF HEARING LOSS

History
- Hearing loss is a common complaint, especially in the elderly. Determining the cause of the hearing loss (conductive, sensorineural or mixed) may direct treatment
- The most common causes of conductive hearing loss are:
  - Otosclerosis (stiffening of the ossicles)
  - Cerumen impaction
  - Otitis media
- Sensorineural hearing loss is frequently due to presbycusis (high frequency hearing loss of aging) or noise exposure. An audiogram will determine the severity and type of hearing loss by measuring the softest sounds (in decibels) the patient can hear. A difference between the air conduction thresholds and bone conduction thresholds suggests a conductive hearing loss. Bone and air thresholds are usually the same in patients with sensorineural hearing loss

Table 3.1: Types of Hearing Loss

	Definition	Cause
Conductive	External or middle ear dysfunction causing impairment of the passage of sound vibrations to the inner ear	- Obstruction such as cerumen impaction - Mass loading (e.g., middle ear effusion) - Stiffness (osteosclerosis) - Discontinuity (ossicular disruption)
Sensory	Detiroration of the cochlea	- Loss of hair cells from the organ of Corti - Noise exposure - Head trauma - Systemic disease
Neural	Lesions involving the 8th CN, auditory nuclei, ascending tracts, or auditory cortex	- Acoustic neuroma - Multiple sclerosis - Auditory neuropathy

Table 3.2: Diagnostic Evaluation

Classification of Hearing Loss	Voice Level	Decibel Range
Normal	Soft whisper	0-20
Mild	Soft spoken voice	21-40
Moderate	Normal spoken voice	41-55
Moderately Severe		56-70
Severe	Loud spoken voice	71-90
Profound	Shout	>90

Physical Exam

Otoscopic Exam
- Evaluate for cerumen impaction, otitis externa, tympanic membrane integrity, and otitis media with effusion

Weber Test
- Place a vibrating 256 Hz tuning fork in the middle of the forehead. A normal patient will not notice a difference in 1 ear versus the other. The sound is louder in the effected ear of a patient with conductive hearing loss. The sound is louder in the normal ear of a patient with sensorineural hearing loss

Rinne Test
- Place a vibrating 512 Hz tuning fork on the mastoid process behind the ear. When ringing is no longer heard, the tuning fork is moved just outside the auditory canal. A normal or positive Rinne test is when the ringing outside the auditory canal is louder than the initial sound heard when the tuning fork is on the mastoid process. A negative Rinne test, or decreased sound outside the auditory canal, indicates conductive hearing loss

Treatment
- Options depend on the etiology of the hearing loss. In conductive hearing loss, treatment is directed at restoring the patency of the auditory canal by cerumen removal, reduction in swelling and treating infectious processes if present. Sensorineural hearing loss is typically treated by reducing background noise, sound amplification devices, and cochlear implants if hearing loss is severe bilaterally

3.2 TINNITUS
- The sensation of sound in the ears, such as ringing or roaring, without external stimulus. It may accompany hearing loss

Cause
- Often caused by damage to the stereocilia, which can release an electrical signal to the auditory nerve that is interpreted as sound. Damage can be caused by age related changes or exposure to loud noise. Objective or pulsatile tinnitus requires imaging studies of the temporal bone for evaluation

Treatment
- Treatment is aimed at reducing annoyance caused by tinnitus and not resolution. It is often masked by using background noise, such as using a hearing aid to introduce a more pleasant noise into the ear

3.3 OTITIS MEDIA AND OTITIS EXTERNA

Otitis Media

- An inflammatory process of the middle ear. It can be classified into acute otitis media (AOM), which can be bacterial or viral and has associated symptoms of fever or pain. Otitis media with effusion (OME) is middle ear fluid without fever or pain

Etiology

- The most common bacterial causes of AOM are *Streptococcus pneumonia, Haemophilus influenza*, and *Moraxella catarrhalis*. OME can develop after an episode of AOM

Presentation

- AOM presents with otalgia, fever, and bulging tympanic membrane. OME includes persistent hearing loss and dull or immobile tympanic membrane

Treatment

- AOM is treated with antibiotic therapy, although observation for fever or progressive symptoms is acceptable for 2 days. Amoxicillin is generally the 1st choice, although ampicillin, amoxicillin-clavulinic acid, or trimethoprim/sulfizoxazole are also acceptable treatments. OME is managed by observation or nasal decongestants. If middle ear fluid persists then tympanostomy tubes can be considered. Untreated AOM will rarely extend into the surrounding soft tissue or the central nervous system leading to meningitis or intracranial abscess

Otitis Externa

- A painful inflammation of the ear canal with purulent ear drainage. Malignant otitis externa is a severe form usually in immunocompromised or diabetic patients that leads to invasion of adjacent bone

Etiology

- *Pseudomonas aeruginosa* is the most common cause of acute otitis externa, although other aerobic Gram Negative species or funguses are other common causes

Presentation

- Acute otitis externa (AOE) presents with fever, irritability, and acute pain, with inflamed ear canal and tenderness of the ear. AOE is commonly called "swimmer's ear" that is contracted from swimming in water contaminated with aerobic Gram Negative species

Treatment

- The commonly indicated bacteria are sensitive to acidic environments so that topical agents with low pH, such as in acetic acid solutions, are most effective. Topical antibiotic solutions may also be used. If the canal is swollen shut, a small foam wick may be placed in the ear canal to allow penetration of the antibiotic drops

3.4 CERUMEN IMPACTION

- Cerumen is a protective wax material secreted by the ear canal
- Most people produce the dominant "sticky" type of ear wax, in which case the ear canal is largely "self-cleaning" unless external factors interfere
- Cerumen impaction can be caused or exacerbated by foreign bodies intended to remove ear wax, however, in actuality, they are causing wax to be pushed further into the ear canal and causing irritation or pain
- Treatment is aimed at gentle removal of the ear wax either by manual disimpaction by a clinician with a curette or water jet irrigator. Hydrogen peroxide solutions with gentle irrigation can also be used at home

3.5 UPPER RESPIRATORY TRACT DISORDERS

Sinusitis

- Inflammation of the sinuses
- Normally ciliary activity clears sinuses of mucus so the sinuses are largely sterile. If the sinuses become obstructed than mucus can accumulate producing signs and symptoms of sinusitis and increasing susceptibility to **sinus infection** by bacteria
- Sinusitis is a very common primary care office complaint and can be classified by its duration (acute or chronic), the etiology, and the pathogen

Acute Rhinosinusitis

- Sinusitis of less than 4 weeks duration—typically it occurs secondary to a viral upper respiratory infection

Etiology

- Sinusitis is caused by obstruction either from infectious causes such as viruses, or non-infectious causes such as allergic rhinitis, barotraumas, and exposure to chemical irritants
- Less common causes of obstruction can occur from polyps, sinus tumors, granulomatous disease, and cystic fibrosis leading to decreased mucus clearance
- Viral sinusitis from common pathogens such as rhinovirus, parainfluenza, and influenza is more common than bacterial causes
- Bacterial sinusitis is most commonly caused by *Streptococcus pneumonia* and *Haemophilus influenza*; however, MRSA is an emerging cause of bacterial sinusitis
- Diabetics and other immunocompromised individuals are more likely to have atypical or polymycrobial infections such as fungal or *Pseudomonas* infections

Presentation

- Most cases of acute sinusitis occur after a viral URI
- Symptoms typically include nasal drainage, congestion, facial pain or pressure, and headache
- Purulent discharge with fever is more common with bacterial sinusitis
- Tooth pain, especially in the upper molars, is more commonly associated with bacterial sinusitis
- Pain may localize to tenderness with palpation over the affected sinuses
- Bacterial sinusitis can be reliably diagnosed in patients with symptoms lasting greater than 10 days

Treatment
- Most cases of acute sinusitis improve without antibiotics. Generally supportive care with decongestants, nasal glucocorticoids, and nasal lavage is preferred in patients with mild to moderate symptoms
- Adult patients who do not improve after 7 days or who have severe symptoms should be started on antibiotics. However, patients with mild to moderate symptoms and duration of symptoms less than 7 days showed that antibiotics had no significant impact on cure rates
- Treatment targeted at the most common pathogens includes antibiotics such as amoxicillin and augmentin
- If severe disease develops or intracranial complications occur, patients should undergo surgical intervention and IV antibiotic administration

Chronic Sinusitis
- The presence of sinus inflammation symptoms lasting more than 12 weeks
- It is increasingly thought that underlying inflammation is the cause of chronic sinusitis more than it being primarily an infectious process
- The natural history of the illness is constant nasal congestion and sinus pressure with intermittent flares
- Patients should have a CT sinus to evaluate for possible structural obstructions such as polyps. Patients should also be evaluated by an otolaryngologist to visualize the sinuses and collect direct cultures
- Antibiotic treatment is directed by culture data and is often a prolonged 3 to 4 week course; however, appropriate treatment with concurrent topical/oral glucocorticoids and mechanical irrigation is important
- Surgery may be indicated if therapy fails

Allergic Rhinitis
- After exposure to an allergen, patients develop allergic rhinitis symptoms
- Approximately 20% of the North American population is affected and may occur in seasonal variations
- It is more common in people with a family history or individuals with a personal history of asthma, eczema, or urticaria
- Symptoms generally present before 40 years of age—symptoms will gradually decline with age

Etiology
- Allergic rhinitis is a Type I allergic reaction with mast cell degranulation. Degranulation occurs after the patient is sensitized by as antigen, develops B-cell memory, and then has a re-exposure. IgA in the mucosal surface is responsible in large part for the rhinorrhea present in allergic rhinitis. The most typical pollen allergens are caused by trees, grasses, and weeds that depend of wind for pollination—these are typical causes of seasonal allergies. Perennial allergies can be caused by animal dander, cockroaches, mold, dust, and dust mites

Presentation
- Patients present with episodic sneezing, rhinorrhea, nasal passage obstruction, itching of the eyes, nose, or throat, and tearing of the eyes. On exam the nasal turbinates appear boggy and pale, conjunctiva is injected, and oropharynx unremarkable. Nasal polyps are sometimes noted

Treatment

- Diagnosis of allergic rhinitis is largely made by history and can identify likely allergens by annual timing of symptoms
- Skin testing can be used to identify specific allergens
- Serum levels of IgE are often elevated
- Treatment is aimed at prevention of symptoms. Avoiding the allergen if possible is the most effective method
- Oral H1 antihistamines (fexofenadine, loratadine, cetirizine, diphenhydramine) assist in managing itching, sneezing, rhinorrhea, and ocular manifestations; however, H1 antihistamines do not treat nasal congestion. Newer H1 antihistamines are more selective and less likely to cause sedation. To treat nasal congestion, topical adrenergic agents such as phenylephrine can be used for the short term, but can cause rebound rhinitis after prolonged use. Oral adrenergic agents such as pseudoephedrine can be used to treat nasal congestion, but also are most effective if used for short term. A leukotriene inhibitor such as montelukast is helpful in treating allergic rhinitis. Intranasal glucocorticoids (e.g.; beclomethasone, fluticasone, budesonide) are the most effective methods of treating nasal congestion, rhinorrhea, and itching

Pharyngitis

- Sore throat caused by either a viral or bacterial infection
- One of the most common presenting complaints in primary care

Etiology

- Pharyngitis is a typical-presenting symptom for respiratory viruses, and viruses are the most common cause of pharyngitis
- Rhinoviruses account for approximately 20% of all acute pharyngitis cases and 5% of all cases are caused by coronaviruses
- Other frequent viral pathogens include influenza, parainfluenza, and adenovirus
- Less common viral causes of pharyngitis include herpes simplex virus 1 and 2, cytomegalovirus, Epstein-Barr virus, and acute HIV infection
- Bacterial pharyngitis accounts for approximately 5 to 15% of all acute pharyngitis cases
- Most cases in adults (5 to 15%) is Group A hemolytic *Streptococcus pyogenes,* which is associated with rheumatic fever and acute glomerulonephritis
- Other causes of strep pharyngitis include Group C and G *Streptococcus* infections, which are non-rheumatogenic
- *Fusobacterium necrophorum* is almost as common as strep pharyngitis and can cause Lemierre's disease, an infectious thrombophlebitis of the jugular vein
- Depending on a patient's exposure, other bacterial agents should be considered such as *Neisseria gonorrhoeae, Corynebacterium diptherieae, Corynebacterium ulcerans, Yersinia enterocolitica, Treponema pallidum* (as seen in secondary syphilis), *Mycobacterium pneumonia*, and *Corynebacterium pneumoniae*

Presentation

- In a viral URI setting, acute pharyngitis, as caused by rhinovirus or cornovirus, is usually mild and associated with other nonspecific URI symptoms such as rhinorrhea, congestion, and cough
- Viral pharyngitis is typically not associated with fever, tender cervical adenopathy, or pharyngeal exudates

- Viral pharyngitis can be severe when caused by influenza or adenovirus and will be associated with fever, myalgias, headache, and cough
- Adenovirus may additionally be associated with conjunctivitis in about 1/3 to 1/2 of patients infected
- More rare causes of viral pharyngitis can be distinguished by physical exam findings
- HSV infection has vesicles and shallow ulcers on the palate, as well as pharyngeal exudates and inflammation
- The small vesicles associated with Coxsackie virus are found on the uvula and soft palate and form small white ulcers after rupture
- Both EBV and CMV can have exudative pharyngitis with fever, fatigue, lymphadenopathy, and enlarged spleen making it difficult to distinguish clinically from acute *Streptococcal* pharyngitis
- In the setting of acute HIV infection, patients frequently develop a flu-like prodrome with myalgias, arthralgias, malaise, fever, pharyngitis, and sometimes a maculopapular rash
- The presentation of bacterial *Streptococcal* pharyngitis is similar in group A, C, and G with a wide variance in severity of symptoms. Patients present with fever, chills, and abdominal pain in addition to the pharyngeal pain, but no cough
  - On exam there is tonsillar enlargement and exudates with tender cervical lymphadenopathy
  - The Centor Criteria are typically used to distinguish *Streptococcal* pharyngitis and determine antibiotic usage. Some strains of *Streptococcal* pyogenes can present with a "strawberry tongue" and erythematous rash
  - Other bacterial causes of pharyngitis typically present with exudates but generally are non-specific in their clinical findings and must be distinguished based on history alone

Treatment
- Determined by the etiology. Viral pharyngitis is managed by supportive care. However, bacterial often requires antibiotic therapy
- Throat swab culture is the gold standard for diagnosis, but rapid-antigen testing can have up to a 90% specificity, although sensitivity is only 65 to 90% depending on clinical presentation and collection technique
- The Centor Criteria is used to raise the sensitivity of testing and determine appropriateness of antibiotic usage. A score of less than 2 points directs against antibiotic usage. A score of 2 to 3 points should receive a throat swab and antibiotic usage dictated by results of culture data. Scores greater than 3 points should empirically be started on antibiotic therapy

Table 3.3: Centor Criteria for Antibiotic Usage

Sign or Symptom	Point Value
History of fever	Add 1
Tonsillar exudates	Add 1
Tender anterior cervical lymphadenopathy	Add 1
Absence of cough	Add 1
Age <15 years	Add 1
Age >44 years	Subtract 1

- Prompt treatment of *S. pyogenes* with antibiotics reduces the risk of rheumatic fever; however, rheumatic fever is a rare sequelae even among untreated patients. Treatment within 48-hours of the onset of symptoms typically reduces the duration of symptoms, as well as reducing the potential spread of disease
- Penicillin IM for 1 dose or PO for 10 days is the treatment of choice for Strep pharyngitis, although erythromycin and azithromycin are commonly used—resistance has been growing to these antibiotics. Complications from failure to treat include rheumatic fever, as noted, and local invasions into the surrounding structures, sometimes with abscess development. Acute glomerulonephritis is another complication, which is not preventable by antibiotic treatment
- In viral pharyngitis, patients suffering from influenza antivirals like oseltamivir, zanamivir, amantadine, or rimantadine started within the 1st 36 to 48 hours of symptoms, which reduces the duration and severity of illness. Oseltamivir and zanamivir are active against both Influenza A and B. HSV infections can be treated by acyclovir, but treatment is typically reserved for immunocompromised patients

3.6 EPISTAXIS

Sinusitis

- This is a common primary care problem of bleeding from the anterior nasal cavity, usually unilaterally. Posterior or bilateral bleed is a matter of medical urgency and should be evaluated immediately

Etiology

- Most commonly caused by nasal trauma such as nose picking, foreign bodies, or nose blowing. Other causes include rhinitis, dry air, nasal septum deviation, atherosclerotic disease, hypertension, neoplasia, cocaine abuse, alcohol use, and Osler-Webb-Rendu syndrome (hereditary hemorrhagic telangectasias)
- A less common cause is anticoagulation
- The most common location is in the anterior septum in a confluence of superficial veins called Kiesselbach plexus

Presentation

- Bleeds are typically unilateral and self limiting. Patients with epistaxis typically have higher blood pressures, but values usually return to normal once bleed has resolved. Laboratory values such as platelet counts and INR can be useful in evaluating cause of an acute bleed

Treatment

- Direct pressure on the site of the bleed for 15 minutes by compression of nares treats the majority of cases
- Nasal packing or pneumatic sealant can also be used to compress bleeding sites difficult to compress externally
- Sitting upwards reduces venous pressure, and leaning forward decreases the amount of blood swallowed
- A topical decongestant such as phenylephrine acts as a vasoconstrictor. Topical cocaine can also be used as both vasoconstrictor and anesthetic. Silver nitrate can be applied topically to cauterize the bleeding site or a patch can be applied

- If bleeding continues or bleed originates in the posterior nasal cavity, an otolaryngology consult for packing and hospitalization for monitoring and pain control is advised
- In the case of life-threatening hemorrhage, surgical intervention such as ligation of the nasal arterial supply or endovascular embolization may be necessary
- Antibiotic coverage for staphylococcal infection is necessary while packing is in place

3.7 ORAL HEALTH

- **Oral infections and ulcers:** The most common oral infections are from periodontal diseases such as gingivitis. The next most common infections include HSV, such as with cold sores or Candidal species
- **HSV:** Can affect the lips, tongue, or buccal mucosa causing irritating and painful vesicles that progress to painful shallow ulcers. Topical antivirals such as acyclovir can be used on cold sores, but primary infections may require PO or IV antivirals depending on extent and host immunocompetency
- **Oral candidiasis or thrush:** Most commonly caused by *Candida albicans*. Thrush is uncommon in immunocompetent adults, although individuals on prolonged glucocorticoids or antibiotics may develop thrush. Patients develop sore throat and burning in the mouth and throat—exam will reveal white plaques. Treatment is typically oral nystatin or fluconazole, although IV formulations can be used in resistant cases
- **Vincent's angina or trench mouth:** Acute necrotizing ulcerative gingivitis with very inflamed, painful gingival and ulcerations of the papillae between teeth that bleed easily. Patients frequently have halitosis from the anaerobic bacterial pathogen causing disease. Other common symptoms are fever, malaise, and lymphadenopathy. Debridement and oral penicillin plus metronidazole or clindamycin is the treatment of choice
- **Ludwig's angina:** A dangerous cellulitis of the sublingual and submandibular spaces that is rapidly progressive. Infection source is typically an infected tooth, especially in the lower jaw. Patients present with a constellation of symptoms including dysphagia, odynophagia, edema, tongue displacement with possible airway obstruction, fever, dysarthria, and drooling. The classic sign is a "hot potato" voice. Patients may require airway protection temporarily with intubation or tracheostomy. Treatment is broad spectrum IV antibiotics such as ampicillin/sulbactam, penicillin, and metronidazole
- **Lemierre's disease:** Or septic thrombophlebitis of the jugular vein can be a complication of *Fusobacterium necrophorum* infection. The deep pharyngeal tissue becomes infected and drains into the lateral pharyngeal space and then the internal jugular vein. Patients typically present initially with pharyngitis, but then neck swelling, stiffness, pain, and dysphagia develop. Sepsis usually develops within a week of sore throat and may develop distant emboli. Mortality is significant. Treat with IV penicillin or clindamycin with concurrent abscess drainage. Anticoagulation is recommended to prevent emboli, but data is not clear on the benefits of anticoagulation therapy

Oral Tumors

- Include tumors from the lips, the hard and soft palate, the tongue, salivary glands, or even the gingiva and oral cavity floor. The anterior 2/3s of the tongue and the floor of the mouth are the most common location for oral tumors

Epidemiology
- Oral tumors are more common in developing countries and represent 3% of new cancer cases in the US
- Squamous cell cancers are the most common, and more than 50% of oral cancers contain oncogenic HPV. HPV-positive oral tumors are typically poorly differentiate, basaloid histopathology, with poor response to chemotherapy and radiation. HPV-16 causes occasional chromosome loss or gross deletions, and show an increased survival after chemoradiotherapy
- Alcohol, age >50 years, and tobacco exposure represent other risk factors for oral tumors, with a heavy prevalence of p53 mutations in alcohol and tobacco users. Smoking is almost exclusively the cause or oral cavity floor, larynx, and hypopharynx cancer

Diagnosis
- Signs and symptoms are associated with local invasion, and will change depending on the location within the oral cavity. Patients may present with swelling, pain, otalgia, dysphagia, odynophagia lasting weeks, and soreness in oral cancers
- Physical examination includes careful inspection of all oral mucosal surfaces, palpation of the tongue, mouth floor, and examining for lymphadenopathy. Most commonly visualized pre-malignant lesions are leukoplakia and erythroplakia. A suspicious lesion should be biopsied for final diagnosis. MRI and CT are useful for staging

Treatment
- Local resection is principally used for localized small tumors. Radiotherapy is utilized as a single treatment for T1 and T2 tumors, almost always including regional lymph nodes. For T1 lesions, control is gained in greater than 90% of cases with radiotherapy, and 70 to 85% of T2 cases gain control
- Tonsillar cancer often has better remission rates as it is detected sooner and can respond to the radiotherapy more readily
- Patients with squamous cell at the tongue base are more difficult to treat as they present later; 75% of patients present with Stage III or IV disease. Chemoradiotherapy is the treatment of choice

Dental Infection
- Dental caries and periodontitis are the sequelae of plaque build-up and bacterial infection leading to the destruction of involved tissues. Plaque is a biofilm composed largely of normal oral bacteria

Dental Caries
- Defined as inclusions in the mineralized tooth from acidic byproducts of bacterial metabolism
- Caries progress inward from the surface, eventually involving the dentin and then the pulp from which infection can extend into the periodontal tissues at the root
- *Streptococcus mutans* is the dominant organism causing caries, but other organisms such as *Lactobacillus acidophilus, Streptococcus salivarius*, and actinomyces also contribute to the formation of dental carries
- Monosaccharides and disaccharides such as glucose, sucrose, lactose, and maltose provide appropriate substrate for glycolysis and contribute to bacterial acid production
- Bacteria can utilize sucrose to synthesize polyglycans that increase adherence and aggregation of bacteria on the tooth surface. This polyglycan can also be utilized

by bacteria as a food source when dietary food sources are absent. This prolongs acid production beyond the period of substrate clearance, increasing the chance of developing dental caries
- Complications of dental caries include extension of infection into the pulp, necrosis of the pulp, extension into the root canal and the periapical area of the periodontal ligament
- Further involvement can result in periapical abscess, nonsuppurating inflammation, or cyst. If the infection goes unchecked, it may result in cellulitis, osteomyelitis, or septic thrombophlebitis (Lemierre's disease)
- Incidence of new dental caries can be affected by 50 to 60% via systemic ingestion of fluoride or 35 to 40% by topical application
- Periodontal disease includes gingivitis and chronic periodontitis, both of which are caused by plaque build-up
- Gingivitis represents an earlier, reversible form of chronic periodontitis. Gingivitis refers to inflammation of the gingiva, or gum line. Onset of disease occurs within 2 weeks of poor tooth hygiene
- Chronic periodontitis, the progression of gingivitis, with permanent bone resorption leads to the loss of tooth support
- Abscess can also develop when chronic inflammations flare at the neck of the tooth in a single location. It accounts for the majority of tooth loss in people older than 35 years
- With periodontal disease there is evidence of inflammatory infiltrate into the gingival, but no direct invasion by bacteria in the early stages
- Gram Negative anaerobic bacteria are predominantly responsible for periodontal disease. Infections are typically microbial and include Porphyromonas gingivalis and Treponema denticola, which grow synergistically

Halitosis

- A foul odor that comes from the nasal passages or oral cavity
- The bacterial decay of food and cellular debris produces sulfur compounds creating the odor
- Halitosis is associated with periodontal disease, dental caries, acute gingivitis, oral abscess, and tongue coating
- Less common causes include esophageal diverticulum with retained food particles, esophageal stasis, sinusitis, lung abscess, and pockets of decay in tonsillar crypts
- There are also systemic diseases that can cause halitosis such as renal failure (ammoniac), hepatic failure (fishy), and ketoacidosis (fruity)
- *Helicobacter pylori* infection can also created ammoniac breath
- Treatment is aimed at correcting poor hygiene including tongue brushing and treating infection

Tongue Syndromes

Glossitis

- A red, smooth surfaced tongue caused by inflammation and subsequent loss of filiform papillae. Typically non-painful, it is often associated with nutritional deficiencies such as niacin, riboflavin, iron, or vitamin E. It may also be caused by drug reactions, dehydration, foods, and even autoimmune reactions. If no cause is identified, empiric nutritional replacement therapy is often the best first-line therapy

Glossodynia

- A painful burning of the tongue which occurs both with and without concurrent glossitis. In the presence of glossitis, it is associated with diabetes, diuretics, tobacco, xerostomia, and candidiasis. "Burning mouth syndrome" is glossodynia without and identifiable cause. Glossodynia is most common in post menopausal women, and is typically benign. If symptoms are unilateral or suggest involvement of a cranial nerve, imaging of the brain is reasonable to identify possible neuropathology. Treatments include alpha-lipoic acid and clonazepam, as well as behavioral therapy

Leukoplakia

- A white lesion that cannot be removed by rubbing. Often they are caused by chronic irritation such as from dentures or tobacco, but about 2 to 6% represent dysplasia or early invasive squamous cell carcinoma. Any enlarging areas of leukoplakia should be biopsied

Erythroplakia

- Similar to leukoplakia, but also have erythema underlying it. 90% of erythroplakia cases are associated with dysplasia or squamous cell carcinoma. Risk factors include alcohol and tobacco use. All erythroplakia lesions should be biopsied

Oral Lichen Planus

- A lacy leukoplakia often with an erosive component caused by chronic inflammatory autoimmune disease. It is present in 0.5 to 2% of the population. Lesions are often difficult to differentiate between lichen planus and infectious or cancerous lesions. Exfoliative cytology or biopsy is indicated if squamous cell carcinoma is suspected, but only about 1% of lichen planus evolves into SCC. Treatment is aimed at reducing inflammation with corticosteroids, cyclosporines, and retinoids

Hairy Leukoplakia

- Slightly raised leukoplakic are on the edge of the tongue with a corrugated surface. It is a common early finding in HIV infection and responds clinically to zidovudine or acyclovir

3.8 TEMPOROMANDIBULAR DISORDERS (TMD)

Sinusitis

- Affects 3 to 7% of the population and is a musculoskeletal disorder affecting the temporomandibular joint, and may include the masticatory muscles
- TMD can be acute, recurrent, or chronic
- Women of childbearing age are more likely to experience TMD, and incidence declines after 55 years

Etiology

- The cause of TMD is multifactorial with genetics, trauma, and stress all playing a part
- TMD is the perpetuated by stress, harmful habits such as clenching or grinding, poor posture, and poor sleep habits. Bruxism, the grinding of teeth during sleep, can simultaneously be a predisposing and perpetuating cause of TMD. However, malocclusion has not been shown to increase TMD incidence

Presentation
- Patients typically present with jaw, face, and head pain. They may have difficulty opening their jaw or experience catching or sticking with accompanying joint popping and clicking
- Global headache, shoulder, and neck pain are also common as well as tooth sensitivity, malocclusion, and abnormal tooth wear
- Occasionally tinnitus, dizziness, and hearing loss are noted
- CT can show bony tissue degenerative changes while MRI can evaluate for soft and hard tissue abnormalities

Treatment
- Conservative management is the most common method of treatment; less than 5% of cases require treatment. A combination of self-care, physical therapy, splinting, and medication with muscle relaxants and NSAIDs can provide significant relief of pain. Short courses of oral steroids and opiates can be used in patients with moderate to severe pain who are not responding to initial therapy; joint injections with steroid can also be useful. Alternative therapy such as massage has also shown beneficial effects

Self-care Recommendations
- The rest of the muscles and joints allow healing
- Soft food enables muscles and joints to heal
- Not chewing gum lessens muscle fatigue and joint pain
- Relax your facial muscles: "Lips relaxed teeth apart"
- No clenching; it irritates joints and muscles
- Yawning against pressure prevents locking open and jaw pain
- Moist heat for 20 minutes promotes healing and relaxation
- Ice is for severe pain and new injuries (less than 72 hours)
- Heat and ice—5 seconds of heat, 5 seconds of ice—for pain relief
- Good posture; avoid head-forward position
- Sleeping position: Side lying, with good pillow support
- Jaw exercise: Open and close against finger pressure
- Exercise: 20 to 30 minutes at least 3 times a week
- Acupressure massage between thumb and forefinger
- Over-the-counter analgesics
- Yoga and meditation for stress reduction
- Massage promotes healing and relaxation
- An athletic mouth guard can give temporary relief
- Avoid long dental appointments
- Do not cradle the telephone—it aggravates the neck and jaw

REFERENCES & SUGGESTED READINGS

1. Johnston C, Harper G, Landefeld C. Chapter 4. Geriatric Disorders. In: Papadakis MA, McPhee SJ, Rabow MW, eds. *CURRENT Medical Diagnosis & Treatment* 2013. New York: McGraw-Hill; 2013.

2. Ropper AH, Samuels MA. Chapter 15. Deafness, Dizziness, and Disorders of Equilibrium. In: Ropper AH, Samuels MA, eds. *Adams and Victor's Principles of Neurology.* 9th ed. New York: McGraw-Hill; 2009.

3. Pai S, Parikh SR. Chapter 49. Otitis Media. In: Lalwani AK, ed. *CURRENT Diagnosis & Treatment in Otolaryngology—Head & Neck Surgery.* 3rd ed. New York: McGraw-Hill; 2012.

4. Ray CG, Ryan KJ. Chapter 59. Eye, Ear, and Sinus Infections. In: Ray CG, Ryan KJ, eds. *Sherris Medical Microbiology.* 5th ed. New York: McGraw-Hill; 2010.

5. Lustig LR, Schindler JS. Chapter 8. Ear, Nose, & Throat Disorders. In: Papadakis MA, McPhee SJ, Rabow MW, eds. *CURRENT Medical Diagnosis & Treatment* 2013. New York: McGraw-Hill; 2013.

6. Rubin MA, Ford LC, Gonzales R. Chapter 31. Pharyngitis, Sinusitis, Otitis, and Other Upper Respiratory Tract Infections. In: Longo DL, Fauci AS, Kasper DL, Hauser SL, Jameson JL, Loscalzo J, eds. *Harrison's Principles of Internal Medicine.* 18th ed. New York: McGraw-Hill; 2012.

7. Austen KF. Chapter 317. Allergies, Anaphylaxis, and Systemic Mastocytosis. In: Longo DL, Fauci AS, Kasper DL, Hauser SL, Jameson JL, Loscalzo J, eds. *Harrison's Principles of Internal Medicine.* 18th ed. New York: McGraw-Hill; 2012.

8. Rubin MA, Ford LC, Gonzales R. Chapter 31. Pharyngitis, Sinusitis, Otitis, and Other Upper Respiratory Tract Infections. In: Longo DL, Fauci AS, Kasper DL, Hauser SL, Jameson JL, Loscalzo J, eds. *Harrison's Principles of Internal Medicine.* 18th ed. New York: McGraw-Hill; 2012.

9. Lustig LR, Schindler JS. Chapter 8. Ear, Nose, & Throat Disorders. In: Papadakis MA, McPhee SJ, Rabow MW, eds. *CURRENT Medical Diagnosis & Treatment* 2013. New York: McGraw-Hill; 2013.

10. Goddard G. Chapter 26. Temporomandibular Disorders. In: Lalwani AK, ed. *CURRENT Diagnosis & Treatment in Otolaryngology—Head & Neck Surgery.* 3rd ed. New York: McGraw-Hill; 2012.

NOTES

4 OPHTHALMOLOGY

Mohamed Abou Shousha, MD

Matthew D. Council, MD

Contents

4.1 BASIC ANATOMY AND FUNCTION

- **Eyelids:** Provide protection to the eye. They evenly spread the tear film on the ocular surface. Eyelid margins carry meibomian glands, which provide an important component of the tear film. Dysfunction of these glands can cause a form of blepharitis and dry eye
- **Conjunctiva:** Lines the inner aspect of the eyelids and covers the sclera. The conjunctiva secretes an important component of the tear film and provides the immune surveillance of the ocular surface
- **Cornea:** It is the transparent avascular anterior surface of the eye. It transmits and focuses light on the photoreceptors of the retina. Minor irregularities or opacities in the cornea can significantly affect visual acuity. The cornea is very densely innervated, and thus corneal diseases such as an abrasion can be associated with severe pain
- **Anterior chamber angle:** It is the angle between the cornea anteriorly and the iris posteriorly and is responsible for draining out the aqueous humor and thus maintaining a normal intraocular pressure. Dysfunction in this area can cause a form of glaucoma
- **Crystalline lens:** Together with the cornea, it focuses incoming light on the photoreceptors of the retina. Contraction of the ciliary muscle surrounding the lens allows accommodation of the lens, the ability to focus on objects at different distances from the eye
- **Uvea:** Composed of the iris, ciliary body and choroid. The iris forms the pupil, which continuously controls the amount of light entering the eye similar to the shutter of a camera. The ciliary body secretes the aqueous humor, which provides nutrition to the avascular cornea and lens. The choroid provides nutrition to the outer layers of the retina
- **Retina:** Has the photoreceptors, which convert light to electrical impulses. The peripheral part of the retina provides night vision and visual field. The central part of the retina, the macula, is the most sensitive part, providing fine central vision
- **Optic nerve:** Carries the electrical impulses from the retina to the brain. The optic nerve head can be visualized during direct ophthalmoscopy and is seen nasal to the macula. The optic nerve is surrounded by the 3 meningeal sheaths of the brain and its subarachnoid space is connected to that of the brain
- **Orbit:** The skull socket, which contains and protects the eye globe, part of the optic nerve, the extraocular muscles, nerves, and blood vessels. The orbital apertures are continuous with the intracranial cavity

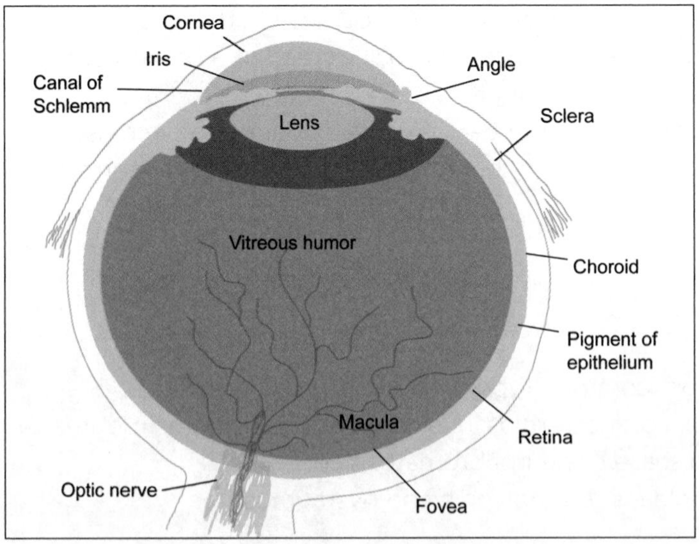

Figure 4.1: Schematic figure of the eye globe

4.2 BASIC EYE EXAMINATION

- Test visual acuity of each eye with the patient's glasses or reading glasses, if available
- Test confrontational visual fields for each eye
- Inspect the eyelids, conjunctiva, sclera, cornea, and iris
- Test the motility of the extraocular muscles
- Assess anterior chamber depth and clarity
- Test the pupils for direct and consensual light reflexes
- Assess the crystalline lens for clarity
- Examination of the fundus using a direct ophthalmoscope

4.3 COMMON CAUSES OF VISUAL LOSS

I- Refractive Errors

Clear vision is achieved by focusing the image of an object on the macula. Failure of this focusing is called refractive error and is the most common cause of reversible decrease in vision. Eyeglasses or contact lenses can correct most of refractive errors. Refractive surgery such as LASIK (laser-assisted in situ keratomileusis) can also be used to correct refractive errors.

- **Amblyopia or lazy eye:** Irreversible decrease of vision in 1 eye secondary to underdevelopment of the visual cortex. Usually caused by uncorrected refractive errors or misalignment of the eyes during childhood. Can be prevented by early screening and intervention
- **Myopia (Nearsightedness):** Blurring of distance vision. Image of the distant object is focused anterior to the macula. Near vision is preserved unless the myopia is severe
- **Hyperopia (Farsightedness):** Blurring of near vision. Image of the distant object is focused posterior to the macula. Far vision is preserved in mild hyperopia. Accommodation can compensate for mild hyperopia but may lead to eye strain and headaches. Compensatory accommodation in children can result in crossed eyes (accommodative esotropia)

- **Astigmatism:** Astigmatism occurs when the curvatures of the cornea (or the lens) at different axes are not equal (the shape of an American football instead of a basketball), resulting in failure to focus the image on the macula
- **Presbyopia:** Progressive age related diminution of near vision secondary to a decrease in the amplitude of accommodation. Usually starts in the 4th decade. Vision is fully corrected by appropriate reading glasses

II- Cataract

Opacification of the crystalline lens.

Types
- Senile (age-related) cataract: The most common type
- Secondary: May be seen with trauma, corticosteroids, uveitis, radiation, diabetes mellitus, or systemic diseases such as Wilson's disease or neurofibromatosis type 2
- Congenital or developmental: Usually leads to amblyopia and nystagmus

Symptoms
- Painless, slowly progressive blurring of vision that is usually bilateral yet often asymmetrical
- Glare (often with bright sun light or automobile headlights at night)
- Decreased color vision
- Some patients initially notice frequent changes in their eyeglass prescriptions and improvement of near vision in a phenomenon known as second sight

Signs
- Decreased visual acuity
- Direct ophthalmoscopy: Clouding of the lens, dim or absent red reflex, difficulty visualizing the retina

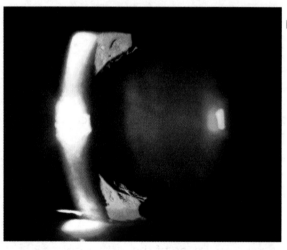

Figure 4.2: Senile cataract

Treatment
- Surgical removal of the lens followed by placement of an intraocular lens
- Surgery is indicated if the decrease in vision affects a patient's ability to perform his/her activities of daily living. The ophthalmologist may sometimes advise earlier or delayed intervention depending on other ocular comorbidities
- Cataract surgery is usually an outpatient surgery

- Anesthesia: MAC (monitored anesthesia care) and topical eye drops with or without local injections of anesthetic agents (intraocular or retro/peri-bulbar injections). General anesthesia is rarely needed. Sedation is sometimes needed in anxious uncooperative patients
- The risk of serious bleeding is low. Discussion of benefit to risk ratio of discontinuing anticoagulation perioperatively must be addressed by the ophthalmologist and the internist. Anticoagulation can often be continued in routine cataract surgeries

4.4 AGE RELATED MACULAR DEGENERATION (AMD)

- AMD is a major global public health problem. 12% of Caucasian males and 16% of Caucasian females older than 80 years in the US suffer from the disease
- It is the leading cause of legal blindness in the elderly Caucasian population in the US. It accounts for around 54% of all cases
- Risk factors are age, Caucasian race, family history, smoking, and hypertension

Types

1- Dry type (atrophic, non-exudative): 90% of cases

Symptoms

- Gradual loss of central vision (usually over months or years)
- Distortion of vision
- An Amsler grid can be used to assess the progression of the disease. It is a grid of horizontal and vertical lines. A change or distortion in the lines may indicate progression of the disease, which may require treatment

Signs

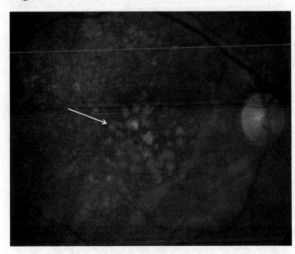

Figure 4.3: Drusen in age-related macular degeneration

- Drusen are small yellow or white spots in the macula. They are usually bilateral but may be asymmetric
- In advanced cases, sharply demarcated areas of retinal atrophy (geographic atrophy) are seen

2- Neovascular or exudative (wet): 10% of cases

Symptoms

- Central visual loss, which may be rapidly progressive

Signs

- Macular drusen, retinal pigment epithelial detachment
- Choroidal neovascularization with retinal hemorrhages
- Subretinal fibrosis and scar

Screening

- A comprehensive eye exam by an ophthalmologist is recommended every 2 years for people under age 65 and annually for those over age 65

Prevention

- A diet rich in leafy green vegetables may lower the risk of AMD
- Cessation of smoking
- Protective measures against exposure to excessive sunlight
- Control of hypertension

Treatment

Dry AMD:

- **High dose antioxidant vitamins and minerals (vitamin C and E, beta-carotene, zinc, and copper – AREDS formula):** Can decrease the risk of AMD progression in moderate and advanced AMD. Note that there is an increased risk of lung cancer with beta-carotene in smokers and ex-smokers
- **Amsler grid:** Should be provided for self-test on a regular basis
- **Low vision aids**
- **Surgery:** Miniature intraocular telescope implantation or macular translocation surgery may be of benefit

Wet AMD:

- **Intravitreal injections of Anti-VEGF (vascular endothelial growth factor):** The current standard of care
- **Intravitreal injections of steroids**
- **Thermal laser photocoagulation** or **photodynamic therapy (PDT)** may sometimes be used

4.5 GLAUCOMA

- Glaucoma is a progressive optic neuropathy characterized by visual field loss and optic disc cupping. It is usually associated with elevated intraocular pressure, which is the key modifiable factor
- Glaucoma is the 2nd leading cause of legal blindness in the US after AMD and the leading cause among African Americans

Primary Open Angle Glaucoma

- Accounts for 74% of all patients with glaucoma
- More than 2.25 million Americans aged 40 years and older have the disease. About 50% of those are undiagnosed
- Risk factors include high intraocular pressure, age, African American race, family history, diabetes, and myopia

Symptoms
- Usually asymptomatic without redness or pain. Headache or eye pain is only present when the pressure is severely elevated
- Loss of peripheral vision
- Central vision is preserved until late in the disease course

Signs
- Visual acuity is likely to be normal except in advanced glaucoma
- Relative afferent pupillary defect indicates substantial progression
- Direct ophthalmoscopy will usually show optic cupping (cup/disc ratio ≥0.5)
- Tonometry shows elevated intraocular pressure
- Perimetry by the ophthalmologist can detect visual field defects

Screening
- Screening is recommended for high-risk groups. A comprehensive eye exam by an ophthalmologist is recommended every 2 years from the age of 45 to 65 and every year afterwards

Treatment
- Medical therapy: Topical prostaglandin analogues, β-blockers, α-2 agonists, carbonic anhydrase inhibitors and/or miotics. These medications may have systemic side effects
- Laser trabeculoplasty: Enhances aqueous outflow and lowers IOP
- Surgical: Trabeculectomy or tube shunt surgeries

Table 4.1: Side Effects of Common Ocular Medications

Medication	Side Effects	Contraindications
β-adrenergic blocking agents	Bronchospasm, bradycardia, hypotension, fatigue, depression, and decreased libido	Asthma and obstructive airways disease, bradycardia, congestive cardiac failure, and 2nd or 3rd degree heart block
α-agonists	Hypotension, dry mouth, dizziness, and fatigue	Children, as the drugs may cross the blood-brain barrier
Prostaglandin analogues	Periocular skin pigmentation, growth of lashes, possible flare of uveitis, or herpetic eye disease	Pregnancy, as animal studies have shown potential teratogenic effects
Oral carbonic anhydrase inhibitors	Paresthesia, fatigue, depression, hypokalemia, acidosis, diarrhea, nausea, aplastic anemia (rare)	Allergy to Sulfa
Corticosteroids	Glaucoma, cataract, and worsening of infections	Infection

Acute Angle-closure Glaucoma
- Occlusion of the trabecular meshwork that drains the aqueous humor out of the eye by the peripheral iris results in a rapid and often severe rise in the intraocular pressure
- High prevalence in individuals of Far Eastern descent

Symptoms
- Haloes around lights, eye pain, and headache
- Precipitating factors include being in a dark room, reading, emotional stress, and medications causing mydriasis such as topical mydriatics, systemic parasympathetic antagonists, or sympathetic agonists (e.g., cold remedies)

Signs
- Reduced vision (often less than 20/200)
- Ciliary hyperemia (violaceous circumcorneal injection) and corneal edema
- Anterior chamber is shallow
- Nonreactive mid-dilated pupil
- Intraocular pressure is usually very high (50 to 100 mmHg)

Treatment
- Immediate referral to an ophthalmologist
- Supine position to encourage the lens to shift posteriorly under the influence of gravity to break the attack
- Systemic: Intravenous acetazolamide, mannitol, or glycerol. Analgesia and an antiemetic may be required
- Topical: α-agonists, β-blockers, steroids, pilocarpine
- Central corneal indentation with an indentation lens can force aqueous into the angle and may break an attack
- In resistant cases: Emergency laser or surgical iridotomy, lens extraction, or trabeculectomy

4.6 DIABETIC RETINOPATHY

- Around 1/3 of diabetics aged 40 years or older have diabetic retinopathy and 4% have vision-threatening complications related to diabetic retinopathy
- More common in type 1 diabetes. Nearly all patients with type 1 diabetes and >60% of patients with type 2 diabetes have diabetic retinopathy during the 1st 2 decades of their disease
- Risk factors: Duration of diabetes (the most important risk factor), poor control of diabetes, hypertension, nephropathy, hyperlipidemia, and smoking. Pregnancy is not a risk factor but can be associated with rapid progression of diabetic retinopathy

Diagnosis

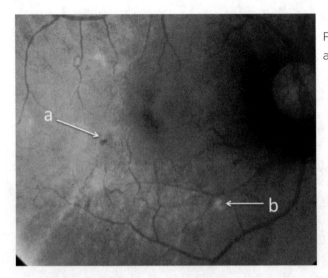

Figure 4.4: Background diabetic retinopathy.
a = blot hemorrhage. b = cotton wool spot

Non-proliferative
- Microaneurysms: Tiny red dots in the retina (the earliest sign)
- Retinal hemorrhages: Flame-shaped and dot/blot hemorrhages
- Exudates: Waxy yellow lesions with relatively distinct margins
- Cotton wool spots: Small, whitish, fluffy superficial lesions

Diabetic Maculopathy
- Macular edema, exudates or ischemia: The most common cause of visual impairment

Proliferative Retinopathy
- Retinal neovascularization: New blood vessels form in response to retinal ischemia. New blood vessels may bleed spontaneously resulting in retinal and vitreous hemorrhages and subsequent retinal fibrosis and detachment
- Iris neovascularization: May cause occlusion of the trabecular meshwork and neovascular glaucoma

Screening
- A dilated comprehensive eye examination by an ophthalmologist is indicated immediately after the diagnosis of diabetes type 2 is made. An examination is indicated within 3–5 years of the diagnosis of type 1 diabetes
- Subsequent examinations for both type 1 and type 2 diabetic patients should be repeated annually. Examinations will be required more frequently if retinopathy is progressing

Treatment
- Improved glycemic and blood pressure control can prevent and delay the progression of diabetic retinopathy
- Laser photocoagulation therapy prevents loss of vision in patients with severe non-proliferative, proliferative diabetic retinopathy and/or macular edema

4.7 ACUTE LOSS OF VISION

Transient Loss of Vision (Amaurosis Fugax)
- **Embolic:** Occlusion of blood supply to the retina or the visual pathway (atrial fibrillation, carotid thrombus)
- **Vasospasm:** Migraine or hypertensive emergency
- **Hypoperfusion:** Low blood pressure, shock, or orthostatic hypotension
- **Functional disorder:** Hysterical and malingering

Sustained Loss of Vision
- **Media opacity:** Corneal edema, hyphema (blood in anterior chamber) and vitreous hemorrhage (e.g., in diabetic retinopathy)
- **Retinal disease:** Retinal detachment, retinal vascular occlusions (e.g., central retinal artery or vein occlusion) and retinal hemorrhages
- **Optic nerve disease:** Optic neuritis (MS, SLE, sarcoidosis), acute glaucoma, ischemic optic neuropathy, and giant cell arteritis
- **Visual pathway disorder:** Stroke

4.8 OCULAR INFECTIONS

Herpes Simplex Keratitis
- The most common infectious cause of corneal blindness in developed countries

Symptoms
- Unilateral discomfort, redness, photophobia, watering, and blurred vision
- Recurrence is common

Signs
- Linear branching (dendritic) corneal ulcer. Often located centrally. Can be seen with fluorescein stain

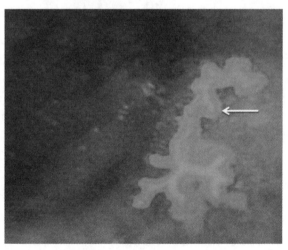

Figure 4.5: Herpetic corneal dendrite (ulcer) stained with fluoroscein

Treatment
- Antiviral eye drops (e.g., topical ganciclovir)
- Most uncomplicated cases resolve by 2 weeks

- Oral antiviral therapy may be indicated, especially in immunodeficient patients
- Topical steroids may exacerbate the keratitis

Herpes Zoster Ophthalmicus

- Shingles involving the V1 dermatome supplied by the ophthalmic division of the 5th cranial nerve (trigeminal). Involvement of the skin of the tip, side and root of the nose correlates strongly with ocular involvement

Presentation

- Acute keratitis: Dendritic lesions
- Can also cause conjunctivitis, episcleritis, scleritis, uveitis, optic neuritis and cranial nerve palsies

Treatment

- Oral antiviral (e.g., acyclovir)
- Systemic steroids: Used only in conjunction with systemic antivirals. Have a moderate effect in reducing acute pain and accelerating skin healing. No effect on the incidence or severity of postherpetic neuralgia

Ocular Manifestations of HIV

HIV Retinal Microangiopathy

- Develops in up to 70% of AIDS patients with declining CD4+ count
  - Symptoms: None
  - Signs: Cotton wool spots and retinal hemorrhages

Cytomegalovirus (CMV) Retinitis

- Is the most common opportunistic ocular infection in AIDS
  - Symptoms: Floaters and blind spots. Up to 50% of patients are asymptomatic
  - Signs: Well-demarcated, geographic, confluent areas of retinal whitening associated with retinal hemorrhages
  - Treatment: Systemic and intravitreal antiviral treatment (e.g., ganciclovir)

Other Ocular Manifestations of AIDS

Kaposi sarcoma, molluscum contagiosum, herpes zoster ophthalmicus, conjunctival squamous cell carcinoma, and progressive outer retinal necrosis.

4.9 EYELID DISEASES

Blepharitis

(see Red Eye Table)

Chalazion

- Chronic, sterile, granulomatous inflammation of the meibomian glands of the eyelid. A secondarily infected chalazion is referred to as an internal hordeolum

Symptoms

- Gradually enlarging painless nodule. Painful if infected

Signs

- A nodule within the eyelid that may be tender if inflamed

Treatment

- Warm compresses: At least a 3rd of chalazia resolve spontaneously
- Persistent lesions may be treated with surgery (incision and curettage) or intralesional steroid injection
- Recurrent chalazia should be biopsied to rule out masqueraders such as sebaceous cell carcinoma of the eyelid

Stye (External Hordeolum)

- An acute staphylococcal abscess of a lash follicle

Diagnosis

- A tender swelling in the lid margin pointing anteriorly, usually with a lash at the apex

Treatment

- Topical antibiotics, hot compresses, and epilation of the associated lash

Eyelid Basal Cell Carcinoma (BCC)

- The most common eyelid malignancy. Slow growing and locally invasive but does not usually metastasize. 90% of basal cells occur in the head and neck and about 10% of these involve the eyelid
- Risk factors: Old age, fair skin, inability to tan, and chronic exposure to sunlight

Presentation

- Firm, pearly nodule with small, dilated blood vessels on the surface

Treatment

- Excision with safety margins. Recurrences after incomplete excisions can be more aggressive

Eyelid Squamous Cell Carcinoma

- Much less common but more aggressive than basal cell carcinoma with metastasis to regional lymph nodes in about 20% of cases

4.10 RED EYE

Table 4.2: Red Eye

	Symptoms	Signs	Management
Subconjunctival Hemorrhage	Mild soreness or foreign body sensation	Unilateral bright red patch under the conjunctiva	None needed
Blepharitis	Usually bilateral ocular discomfort and irritation. Burning, crusting of lashes; worse in morning with remissions and exacerbations	Scales and crusting around lashes Hyperemic and greasy anterior lid margins Capping of meibomian gland orifices with oil globules	Warm compresses and eyelid scrubs Oral tetracyclines Topical antibiotics and steroids
Keratoconjunctivitis sicca (dry eye)	Foreign body sensation, burning, tearing. Typically worse at end of day	Schirmer test with reduced tear production Corneal fluorescein staining shows fine diffuse erosions	Artificial tears Punctual occlusion Topical cyclosporine
Viral conjunctivitis	Excessive watery discharge, irritation, pruritus. Usually starts unilateral then becomes bilateral	Follicles on conjunctival lining of the eyelid Preauricular lymphadenopathy Sometimes associated with sore throat	Supportive (e.g., artificial tears) Avoid close contact with people for 7 to 14 days
Bacterial conjunctivitis	Thick purulent discharge, irritation, pruritus. Unilateral or bilateral	Mucopurulent discharge Sticking of the eye lashes together	Topical antibiotics. Most common organism: *S. pneumoniae*, *S. aureus*, and *H. influenza*
Allergic conjunctivitis	Clear discharge, pruritus. Bilateral	Watery discharge Papillae (red dots) on the conjunctival lining of the eyelid	Topical antihistamine/ mast cell stabilizers
Corneal abrasion	Pain, photophobia, watering, blurred vision. Unilateral	Corneal staining with fluorescein	Prophylactic antibiotic eyedrops or ointment
Episcleritis	Redness and tenderness. Usually unilateral	Inflammation of superficial episcleral vessels	Topical steroid or oral NSAID
Scleritis	Deep aching eye pain	Inflammation of deep episcleral vessels. Scleral Nodule	Periocular steroid injections, systemic steroids, and/or systemic immunosuppressive agents
Uveitis	Pain, photophobia, blurred vision, floaters	Ciliary (circumcorneal) injection which has a violaceous hue Cell and flare in the anterior chamber Hypopyon (settling of cells in the inferior part of the anterior chamber) in severe cases	Topical, periocular and systemic steroids Immunosuppresive agents Work up to determine cause

Other causes of red eye: Foreign body in the eye, pinguecula, pterygium, thyroid-related eye disease, eyelid malposition, keratitis (herpetic, bacterial), acute angle-closure glaucoma

4.11 EYE IN RHEUMATOLOGICAL DISEASES

Table 4.3: Eye in Rheumatological Diseases

Keratoconjunctivitis sicca (dry eye)	Sjögren's syndrome, rheumatoid arthritis, systemic lupus erythematosus, polyarteritis nodosa, scleroderma
Episcleritis and Scleritis	Rheumatoid arthritis, systemic lupus erythematosis, Wegener's granulomatosis, polyarteritis nodosa, relapsing polychondritis
Uveitis	Sarcoidosis, seronegative spondyloarthropathies, Bęhcet disease, Lyme disease, juvenile rheumatoid arthritis
Keratitis	Systemic lupus erythematosis, Wegener's granulomatosis, polyarteritis nodosa
Anterior ischemic optic neuropathy	Giant cell arteritis

4.12 OCULAR EMERGENCIES

Retinal Artery Occlusion

Occlusion of the central retinal artery or one of its branches with a thrombus or embolus.

Symptoms
- Sudden and profound painless loss of vision in 1 eye
- Vision loss can be confined to a sector of the visual field in cases with branch artery occlusion
- Spontaneous dislodgment of the embolus can occur resulting in regaining of vision (amaurosis fugax). This is a form of transient ischemic attack (TIA)

Signs
- Narrowing of the retinal arteries and veins with segmentation of the blood column
- "Cherry red spot" at the center of the fovea is seen surrounded by cloudy white ischemic retina
- Emboli can sometimes be seen

Treatment
The aim is to dislodge the emboli before retinal infarction occurs.
- Ocular massage, intravenous mannitol, sublingual isosorbide dinitrate, topical apraclonidine, topical timolol and intravenous acetazolamide
- STAT ophthalmology consultation
- Anterior chamber paracentesis by an ophthalmologist
- Intra-arterial thrombolysis
- Note that the risk of stroke is high. Stroke workup and prophylaxis is advisable

Acute Angle Closure Glaucoma

1. Eye Trauma
Chemical burns to the eye (EMERGENCY!!)
- **Requires emergency treatment before completing a thorough history and examination.** Alkali burns are the most serious as alkali causes denaturation of proteins and rapidly penetrates into the eye. The most commonly involved alkalis are ammonia, sodium hydroxide, and lime

Immediate treatment
- **Copious irrigation** with sterile normal saline or lactated Ringer's is crucial until pH is neutral (use tap water if necessary to avoid delay). This will often take several liters of fluid
- The speed and efficacy of irrigation is the most important prognostic factor
- A topical anesthetic prior to irrigation improves comfort and facilitates cooperation
- Eversion of the upper eyelid is imperative to identify and remove any retained particles
- STAT ophthalmology consultation

2. Corneal Foreign Body or Abrasions

Symptoms
- Sudden eye discomfort, tearing and photophobia. History suggestive of a foreign body is usually elicited

Signs
- Careful slit lamp exam and fluorescein staining of the cornea to detect the foreign body
- Eversion of the upper eyelid may be necessary to reveal hidden foreign bodies

Treatment
- Foreign body can be removed with a 25 gauge needle held parallel to the cornea under the slit lamp microscope
- Prophylactic antibiotic eye drops are advisable
- Foreign bodies from grinding metals raise suspicion for an intraocular foreign body/ruptured globe. A CT scan of the orbit and ophthalmology consult are advisable in such cases

3. Hyphema

Hemorrhage into the anterior chamber of the eye.
- Symptoms: Blurry vision after a severe blunt trauma
- Signs: Red blood cells sediment inferiorly in the anterior chamber with a resultant "fluid level"
- Treatment is aimed at prevention of secondary hemorrhage and control of any elevation of intraocular pressure. Ophthalmology consult is required. An occult ruptured globe must be ruled out

4. Ruptured Globe
- Caused by penetrating as well as severe blunt trauma
- Prolapse of intraocular structures such as the lens, iris, vitreous, or retina is usually evident
- Note that an anterior rupture may be masked by extensive subconjunctival hemorrhage
- An occult posterior rupture can be associated with little damage to the anterior segment but should be suspected if there is an asymmetry of the anterior chamber depths in the setting of trauma
- Cover the eye with a protective eye shield and get STAT ophthalmology consultation
- Consider CT orbit to rule out intraocular and/or intraorbital foreign bodies, especially if the nature of the injury is suggestive
- Antiemetic as needed to prevent worsening of rupture

NOTES

5 Gynecology & Women's Health

Anne Davis, MD

Contents

5.1 SEXUALITY

Sexual Functioning

- Most women describe themselves as heterosexual, about 4% as bisexual, and about 2% as lesbian; however, about 12% of women report sexual experience with another woman
- Most heterosexual women in the US begin having vaginal intercourse around age 17; 98% of women will have intercourse at least once
- Most couples are satisfied with their sexual relationships and report sex from a few times a week to a few times a month. Even those having sex much less frequently can report high sexual satisfaction
- Important components of the sexual response (desire, arousal, and orgasm) are similar in women and men, but may not occur in a linear manner. For example, many women experience arousal before desire

Low Interest in Sex

- Low interest in sex is common and is only a problem if associated with distress
- Decreased desire may be related to depression or anxiety, co-existing medical illnesses, life stresses, relationship, sexual boredom, or sexual pain
- Medications that can decrease interest in sex include SSRIs and anti-hypertensives, among others. There is no clear link between hormonal contraception and libido
- There is no strong relationship between endogenous testosterone and libido in women

Low Arousal and Difficulty With Orgasm

- As with desire, low arousal and problems with orgasm are only a problem if associated with distress. Sexual satisfaction in women is not tightly linked to the occurrence of orgasm
- Poor sexual stimulation is a common cause of low arousal and lack of orgasm; this can be addressed through couple communication
- Medications interfering with libido can also lead to problems with arousal and orgasm

Pain During Sex (Dyspareunia)

- External pain can be caused by urogenital atrophy after menopause, vaginitis, low arousal, vestibulitis, or vaginismus (muscular tightening of the vaginal opening)
- Internal pain has many causes related to pelvic pathology. Common sources include ovarian cysts, myomas, surgical scarring, and endometriosis

Treatment of Sexual Problems

- In most cases sexual problems improve, but may not resolve, with supportive counseling from a primary care provider or therapist
- No pharmacotherapy has been approved for low libido in women
- Decreased estrogen in menopause can hinder arousal in some women if urogenital atrophy causes dryness and decreased tissue elasticity. These changes can be treated with lubricants and estrogen replacement, either local or systemic
- Pain should be addressed through treatment of its source

5.2 CONTRACEPTION

- More couples need access to effective contraception; half of all pregnancies in the US are unplanned
- The most effective methods are sterilization, which is permanent, and long-acting reversible contraception (LARC) methods of the IUD and implants
- LARC methods have failure rates of less than 1% per year. Methods such as pills, rings, patches, and injections require daily, weekly, or monthly effort by the user as well repeat visits to a pharmacy. With typical use, these methods are associated with pregnancy rates 20 times higher than sterilization or LARC
- Effective contraception is especially important for women with medical conditions that increase maternal and fetal risk with pregnancy; such pregnancies have better outcomes when planned

Combined Hormonal Methods: Pill, Patch, Ring

- Oral contraceptives (OCs) are the most commonly used method in younger women in the US. Women after 35 most often rely on sterilization. There are many OC formulations available. Most OCs contain a synthetic estrogen and progestin; 1 OC contains only a progestin. OCs vary in their doses of estrogenic and progestin doses. Currently available OCs with varying doses have comparable safety profiles
- OCs prevent pregnancy primarily by preventing ovulation. All combined methods (estrogen plus progestin) are immediately reversible, baseline fertility returns completely after only a few weeks
- OCs have at least 3 weeks of active pills and 1 week or fewer of placebo pills (or pill free interval). Bleeding occurs during use of the placebos or pill-free interval. OCs can be taken safely with a pill-free interval every few months or without a pill-free interval (continuously)
- OCs can be started without a back-up method during the 1st 7 days after spontaneous menses begins. If started at some other time, a pregnancy test should be performed and if negative OCs may be started with a back-up method such as condoms for 1 week. OCs given inadvertently in early pregnancy are not harmful because contraceptive steroids are not teratogenic. If a pill is missed, 2 pills may be taken the next day without reducing efficacy
- The contraceptive ring combines an estrogen and progestin and is placed in the vagina for 3 weeks. It is removed and a new ring is placed 1 week later. The contraceptive patch combines an estrogen and progestin and is worn on the skin, 1 week per patch for 3 weeks of the month; it too is removed for a week then restarted with a new patch

Side Effects

- Many women experience some unpredictable, or breakthrough, bleeding in the 1st months of use with OCs, patches and rings which usually resolves. Combined hormonal methods do not cause weight gain or clinically important psychological changes

Table 5.1: Drug Interactions

Medicines that can decrease the efficacy of hormonal contraception
Griseofulvin
Rifampin
Carbamazepine
Phenobarbital
Dilantin
Oxcarbazepine
Bosentan

Safety

- Combined hormonal contraceptives are much safer than pregnancy. Serious complications of use are largely related to thrombotic effects of estrogens

> **Safety of contraception for women with medical conditions: Where to go to know**
>
> U.S. Medical Eligibility Criteria for Contraceptive Use, 2010
> Adapted from the World Health Organization Medical Eligibility Criteria for Contraceptive Use, 4th edition
> www.cdc.gov

- Users experience a very small absolute risk of venous thrombosis, embolism, stroke or myocardial infarction. These risks increase for women who smoke and use methods with estrogens, more dramatically after age 35, and women with a personal or family history of thrombosis, hypertension, personal history of stroke or MI, diabetes with vascular disease, migraine with aura, SLE with vascular disease, cardiac disease or smoking after age 35 years
- Other contraindications include active gallbladder disease, liver dysfunction, and hormonally sensitive cancers (breast, endometrial). Combined methods are not contraindicated for women with a family history of breast cancer
- Use of OCs reduces the risk of ovarian and endometrial cancer, improves acne, decreases menstrual bleeding and dysmenorrhea, lowers risk of PID, and prevents some forms of ovarian cysts

Progestin Only Methods: Injectable and Implants

- Depo-medroxyprogesterone acetate (DMPA) is administered IM every 3 months. The contraceptive implant is a 3 cm flexible rod placed subdermally in the upper arm for 3 years. Both methods have a failure rate of less than 1% per year
- Erratic bleeding is normal with injectable DMPA or the implant. With DMPA bleeding decreases dramatically; 75% of women report amenorrhea after 1 year
- DMPA is associated with weight gain of approximately 5 pounds per year. Implant use is not associated with weight gain. DMPA, but not the implant, causes small, reversible decreases in bone density
- Full return to fertility occurs immediately after implant removal, but may not occur until 18 months after DMPA
- Because progestin-only methods are not pro-thrombotic they are safe when estrogen is contraindicated due to thrombosis risk. For instance, DMPA and implants can be used in women with a history of VTE. Highly-effective methods are essential for women anti-coagulated with coumadin, a potent teratogen

Intrauterine Devices

- Two intrauterine devices are available. The T380A (Copper) IUD contains no hormones and may be used for 10 years. The levonorgestrel IUD elutes a progestin for 5 years
- Both types of IUD prevent fertilization because copper is spermicidal and progestins change cervical mucous to stop sperm penetration
- The copper IUD may cause longer, heavier menses or more cramping, however, in many women their menses does not change. After an initial period of erratic bleeding, the LNG IUD reduces menstrual flow substantially
- After removal, full fertility returns with both devices. The modern IUD does not increase the risk of pelvic inflammatory disease or tubal infertility
- Women who have never been pregnant may safely use either IUD

Barrier Methods

- Male latex condoms are widely used for contraception and are easy obtained over the counter. Polyurethane condoms are as effective as latex versions. Female condoms are also available
- Condom use reduces, but does not eliminate, the risk of STI acquisition
- Typically, at least 15% of couples that use condoms as their only method will experience a pregnancy during a year
- Other barrier methods include the female diaphragm and cervical cap. These methods must be used with a spermicide. Failure rates are high, about 20% per year

Emergency Contraception

- Emergency, or post-coital, contraception reduces the risk of pregnancy after intercourse primarily by inhibiting ovulation. Women over 17 may obtain EC without a prescription
- EC contains progestin in a dose higher than OCs, without estrogen, and will reduce the risk of pregnancy related to unprotected intercourse in the previous 72 hours
- A newer form of EC, ulipristal acetate, is effective for 5 days after unprotected sex
- A copper IUD is effective for EC up to 7 day after unprotected sex

5.3 VAGINITIS

Women with vaginitis describe symptoms with some combination of abnormal discharge, irritation or itching, odor and occasionally pain. Some forms of vaginitis are due to sexually transmitted infections. A directed physical exam and wet preparation should guide diagnosis and treatment. Asymptomatic yeast or BV detected by PAP testing or exam does not require treatment.

Yeast Vaginitis or Vulvitis

- Symptoms: Cheesy or curdy white vaginal discharge and itching, can be intense
- Predisposing factors: Immunosuppression, recent antibiotics
- Exam: Erythematous vulva or vagina, white curdy discharge
- Wet mount: Many WBCs, hyphae on KOH prep, pH is low
- Not sexually transmitted
- Treatment: Oral or topical anti-fungal, latter is OTC

Bacterial Vaginosis
- Symptoms: Discharge, fishy odor especially after intercourse
- Pre-disposing factors: Previous BV, tends to recur
- Exam: Thin, grey vaginal discharge
- Wet mount: + odor with KOH added, Clue cells on saline prep, pH high
- Not sexually transmitted
- Oral or topical metronidazole, avoid alcohol with oral form

Trichomoniasis
- Symptoms: Itching, can be intense
- Predisposing factors: New partner
- Exam: Greenish, frothy vaginal discharge, erythematous vagina and cervix (strawberry cervix)
- Wet mount: WBCs, motile flagellated trichomonads, pH is high
- Treatment: Oral metronidazole 1 dose, also for partner
- Sexually transmitted

Herpes
- Symptoms: Focal edema, pain and vesicles that ulcerate, primary infection may occur with fever and adenopathy
- Predisposing factors: New partner
- Exam: Swollen, tender area on perineum, cervical, labial or perineal blisters or ulcers, vaginal discharge
- Wet mount: WBCs, pH is low
- Treatment: Oral acyclovir or valacyclovir
- Sexually transmitted, symptoms may be due to primary or recurrent HSV

Atrophic Vaginitis
- Symptoms: Painful intercourse, irritation with urination, discharge, itching
- Predisposing factors: Menopause
- Exam: Thinned vulvar tissues, narrowed introitus, erythema
- Wet mount: WBCs
- Treatment: Lubricants, systemic or topical estrogen replacement

5.4 BREAST PAIN (MASTALGIA)
- Breast pain can be cyclical or non-cyclical. Most women with breast pain do not have cancer, but cancer can present with breast pain. Any woman who presents with a breast complaint should have a complete exam of both breasts and axillae
- Cyclical breast pain is usually hormonal in etiology, bilateral, begins in the luteal phase and dissipates with menses. This pain is usually mild but can be stronger
  - Cyclic mastalgia with a normal exam can be treated with a well-fitting bra, warm or cold packs, acetaminophen, or NSAIDs
- Non-cyclical pain is more likely to be unilateral, related to a breast or chest wall lesion. Breast-related causes include: Large breasts, hormone replacement therapy, pregnancy, ductal ectasia, breast cancer, especially inflammatory, mastitis (usually in lactating women), and surgical scarring. The etiology will guide treatment

5.5 BREAST MASS

- In most women who present with a breast mass there is no underlying cancer. Every woman who presents with a breast mass should have a complete exam and if needed, imaging. Breast cancer is strongly related to age. Abnormal physical findings are more likely to indicate cancer in older women and in women with a family history of breast cancer
    - Physical findings suggestive of malignancy include skin changes (peau d'orange, retraction), a mass, nipple ulceration or bloody nipple discharge. Lymphadenopathy may also be present
    - Galactorrhea is not associated with cancer and is usually bilateral
    - Cancerous lesions are more likely to be isolated, hard, irregular, and fixed
- Benign masses: These are most commonly fibroadenomas and cysts
- Imaging: A diagnostic mammogram should be the first test ordered in women over 30 with a new breast mass. Targeted ultrasound, combined with mammography, may aid in evaluation of a breast mass in a woman over 30. Ultrasound is the first step to evaluate a mass in a woman under 30
- As yet, there is no clear role for MRI in the diagnostic evaluation of breast lesions
- A suspicious finding on physical exam should be evaluated for biopsy, even if a diagnostic mammogram is negative

5.6 ABNORMAL UTERINE BLEEDING

- Most women have a menstrual cycle of 21 to 35 days in length, bleeding lasts on average for 5 days, and usual blood loss per cycle is less than 80 mL. Disorders of the menstrual cycle include absence of menstrual bleeding (amenorrhea), fewer menses than normal (oligomenorrhea), bleeding between menses (intermenstrual bleeding) or heavy menstrual bleeding. The work-up of irregular or heavy bleeding should include cervical cytology and endometrial sampling to rule out cancer in women over 35. Ultrasonography is helpful for anatomic causes
- Amenorrhea can be primary—never experiencing a period—or secondary when periods disappear after establishment of menses
    - Primary amenorrhea may be a normal variant in adolescents who start menarche later
    - Secondary amenorrhea and oligomenorrhea: Pregnancy should be ruled out first. Common causes include endocrinopathies such as PCOS, thyroid disorders, hyperprolactinemia, low BMI, vigorous sustained exercise. Premature ovarian failure is an uncommon but important cause and is diagnosed by elevated gonadotropins (FSH)
    - Thyroid disorders can lead to a variety of menstrual disorders, from amenorrhea to heavy, frequent menses with anemia
    - Hyperprolactinemia, from adenomas or medications, can cause oligomenorrhea and amenorrhea. Galactorrhea is often present with bilateral milky white breast discharge

Intermenstrual Bleeding

- Occurs between regular menstrual cycles. Rule out pregnancy. Other causes include cervical or endometrial polyps, myomas, cervicitis (chlamydial is common), endometrial hyperplasia or cancer, or cervical dysplasia/cancer

Heavy Menstrual Bleeding (HMB)

- May lead to severe anemia. A complete blood count should be included. Start iron empirically
- Can be due to endocrinopathies, hemoglobinopathies, or anatomic causes
- Endocrinopathies include hypothyroidism and PCOS. Von Willebrand disease is the most common inherited coagulopathy
- Anatomic causes include uterine polyps and myomas (especially when impinging on the uterine cavity-submucous)

Treatment

- Amenorrhea and oligomenorrhea treatment will depend on the etiology such as correction of thyroid disease and hyperprolactinemia. Primary ovarian failure requires hormone replacement and careful discussion of fertility implications. Menstrual irregularities due to PCOS can be managed with weight loss and OCs in women not seeking pregnancy

> **Polycystic ovarian syndrome (PCOS)**
> Associated with infrequent, irregular and sometimes heavy menstrual flow due to anovulation. Diagnosis: Typical ovarian appearance on sonography, clinical evidence of hyperandrogenism such as hirsutism and acne, with menstrual irregularity. Many patients are also obese and abnormalities of lipids and insulin resistance may be present. Infertility may occur.

- HMB should be treated initially with iron replacement. When not associated with a hormonal etiology or cancer, HMB can be treated with non-hormonal treatments such tranexamic acid, or NSAIDs or hormonal treatments such as OCs, DMPA or the hormonal IUD. Surgical treatments include endometrial ablation, myomectomy or hysterectomy

5.7 DYSMENORRHEA

Dysmenorrhea refers to pain with menstrual bleeding. Primary dysmenorrhea is pain in the absence of an anatomic cause. Primary dysmenorrhea is very common in young women; 85% of adolescents experience menstrual pain and 15% describe it as severe.

- Primary dysmenorrhea: May be associated with nausea, vomiting, and inability to participate in normal activities. Related to over-production of uterine prostaglandins. Effective treatments include NSAIDs, acetaminophen, and hormonal therapy with OCs, DMPA
- Secondary dysmenorrhea may also respond to NSAIDs, acetaminophen, and hormonal treatments; however, when due to another etiology that must be addressed: Myomas, endometriosis

Table 5.2: OTC Pain Relievers for Dysmenorrhea

For treatment of primary symptoms
Ibuprofen
Naproxen sodium
Acetaminophen
Recommend labeled dosing of OTC analgesics

5.8 MENOPAUSE

Menopause is defined as the absence of spontaneous menses for 1 year. The average age at menopause is 50 years old in the US.

- The diagnosis is clinical. FSH levels are elevated in menopause. Perimenopause can be a process of several years normally associated with dramatic hormonal fluctuations; hormonal testing is not helpful
- Most common symptoms are hot flushes/night sweats and vaginal dryness. Not all women get hot flushes, but this is the most bothersome symptom. Other changes: Decreased bone density and long-term increased risk of fracture

Replacement Therapy: Treatment of Symptoms: Systemic

- For women with a uterus, estrogen must be given with a progestin to protect against endometrial hyperplasia and cancer. For women without a uterus, estrogen can be given alone
- Systemic estrogens: Give continuously via transdermal, oral, vaginal ring, cream routes. Start with lowest dose and work your way up for symptoms
- Progestins: Use continuously, use recommended doses via oral or transdermal routes
- Estrogens and progestins are available separately in or combination products
- Estrogens reduce hot flushes and vaginal dryness by 90%, alternatives that do not work as well but are better than placebo include clonidine, progestins alone, SSRI, or gabapentin
- No clear guidelines on how long to continue, try to taper off when patient ready

Replacement Therapy: Treatment of Vaginal Symptoms: Local

- Vaginal pills (estradiol 10 mg twice a week) or 1/2 g cream can be used without increase risk of systemic risks, safe with personal hx breast cancer

Indications

- Symptomatic hot flushes or vaginal dryness, not prevention of heart disease or osteoporosis

Contraindications

- Elevated risk of CVA, MI, DVT, current breast cancer any age, active liver disease (local therapy in vagina likely acceptable risk in any of these conditions)

Risks

- Different for women in their 50s and women 60 and older
  - Younger women estrogen only (no uterus): No increased risk of breast cancer, very small increase VTE, increased risk of heart disease and stroke very small, if any
  - Younger women estrogen and progestin (with uterus): Estrogen and progestin very small increased risk of breast cancer after 4 to 5 years of use. Small increase risk VTE, risk of heart disease and stroke very small if any
  - Older women: Increase risk VTE, MI, CVA as well as breast CA. Absolute risks for all outcomes low but serious outcomes. Higher threshold to start replacement

NOTES

6 **Dermatology**

Adam Friedman, MD, FAAD

Lorraine Rosamilla, MD, FAAD

C o n t e n t s

6.1 COMMON DIAGNOSTIC TESTS

Table 6.1: Dermatologic Diagnostic Examinations

Test	Diagnosis
Tzanck	Herpes virus, Langerhans cells (useful for Langerhans cell histiocytosis)
KOH	Fungi or yeast
Cultures	Bacterial or viral
Gram Stain	Bacteria, eosinophils (useful for erythema toxicum neonatorum)
Patch	Allergic contact dermatitis (ACD)
Mineral Oil preparation	Scabies (mite, feces, ova)
Biopsy	
Shave	Epidermal processes: Includes but not limited to seborrheic keratoses, basal cell carcinoma, squamous cell carcinoma, cutaneous T-cell lymphoma (looking for atypical lymphocytes in the epidermis)
Punch	Includes but not limited to sarcoidosis, granuloma annulare, metastatic cancer
Wedge	Deep processes (panniculitis, deep fungal infections)
Excisional	Dysplastic nevi, melanoma

6.2 COMMON DERMATOSES

Eczematous

Atopic Dermatitis

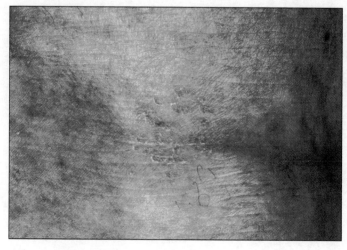

Figure 6.1: Flexural fissured erythematous plaque of eczema

- Major features
  - Pruritus
  - Facial and extensor involvement in infants and children
  - Flexural lichenification (increased skin markings) in adults

- ∘ Chronic or relapsing dermatitis
- ∘ Personal/family history of atopy
- Eye findings: Keratoconus may be associated, anterior and posterior cataracts (usually secondary to long term steroid use)
- Infections
  - ∘ Eczema herpeticum

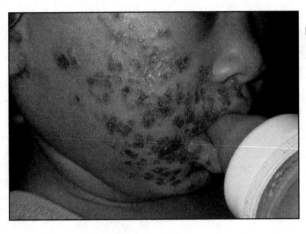

Figure 6.2: Eczema herpeticum

- ∘ Molluscum contagiosum
- ∘ HPV
- ∘ T. rubrum and P. ovale
- ∘ S. aureus in 90%
  - Impaired innate antimicrobial peptides
  - Human B-defensin and cathelicidins – Decreased in AD patients
    - − May explain increased colonization
- Elevated IgE
- Most AD patients DO NOT have food allergy

Contact Dermatitis

- Florist dermatitis - Compositae – Sesquiterpene lactone
  - ∘ Causes: Ragweed, chrysanthemum, feverfew, liverwort, lettuce, sage, artichoke, marigold, sunflower, philodendron, Peruvian lily, and others
  - ∘ Patch test with Sesquiterpene lactone mix
- Chromium
  - ∘ Cement and tanned leather
  - ∘ "Blackjack" felt dermatitis
  - ∘ Cross-reacts with nickel
- Cobalt
  - ∘ Vitamin B12 injections
  - ∘ Cross-reacts with nickel
- Colophony – Resin from tree sap used for adhesion
  - ∘ Bandages
  - ∘ Turpentine lacquer and varnish
  - ∘ Mascara, chewing gum, and newspapers
- Preservatives
  - ∘ Quaternium-15 – #1 cause of preservative dermatitis
  - ∘ Imidazolidinyl urea – #2 culprit

- ○ Quaternium-18-bentonite - "ivy block"
- ○ Parabens
  - • Most common preservative overall
- ○ Glutaraldehyde
  - • Cold sterilizing agent → healthcare workers
- • Latex
  - ○ Cross-reactions
    - • Avocado, banana, chestnut most commonly – Kiwi, passion fruit, mango, fig, cantaloupe, and others
  - ○ Cerebral palsy patients commonly have latex allergy
  - ○ Chemicals that penetrate latex gloves
    - • Nickel, cobalt, formaldehyde, acrylates, epoxy resin, thioglycollate, glutaraldehyde
- • Nickel
  - ○ Dimethylglyoxime test to check for nickel (turns metal pink)
- • Poison ivy/oak: Toxicodendron sp.
  - ○ Pentadecylcatechol from oleoresin or urushiol
  - ○ Cross reactions
    - • Cashew; lacquer tree; mango rind (not juice); Indian marking tree; gingko leaves (not the supplement); Brazilian pepper; Rengas tree (black varnish)

Stasis Dermatitis

- • Subacute to chronic dermatitis with hemosiderin (brown), dilated capillaries in fibrotic dermis
- • May be exacerbated by application of topical steroids or topical antibiotics if a concomitant allergic contact dermatitis is present
- • Often confused for cellulitis ("bilateral cellulitis of the leg" is usually stasis dermatitis)

Pigmented Purpuras

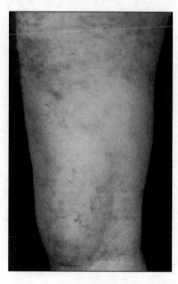

Figure 6.3: Schamberg's pigmented purpura

- • Chronic capillaritis; superficial vessels dilated with endothelial cell hypertrophy and surrounding extravasated red blood cells
- • Variants include:
  - ○ Progressive pigmentary dermatosis of Schamberg

- ◦ Lichen aureus
- ◦ Eczematoid purpura of Doucas and Kapetanakis
- ◦ Lichenoid dermatitis of Gougerot and Blum
- ◦ Purpura annularis telangiectodes of Majocchi

Lichen Planus (LP)

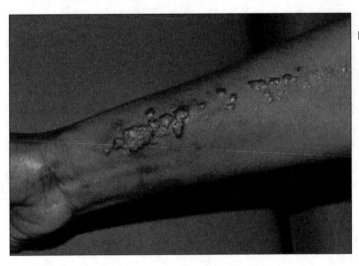

Figure 6.4: Lichen planus

- Inflammatory disorder that affects the skin, mucous membranes, nails, and hair
- The Ps: Purple, polygonal, pruritic, papule, planar
- Wickham's striae – fine, whitish reticulated networks on surface of well-developed plaques
- Prevalence: <1%, no racial preference
- Many clinical subtypes:
    - ◦ Annular (more common in darker skin), atrophic, linear, erosive, hypertrophic (shins)
        - • Erosive mucous membrane disease more common in patients with hepatitis C infection
- Graham-Little syndrome
    - ◦ Follicular lichen planus of skin and/or scalp
    - ◦ Multifocal cicatricial alopecia of scalp
    - ◦ Nonscarring alopecia of axillary and pubic areas
- LP of the nails
    - ◦ 10 to 15% of cases
    - ◦ Usually in combination with other LP lesions on skin
    - ◦ 20-nail dystrophy (trachyonychia)
    - ◦ Thinning, longitudinal ridging, and distal splitting of nail plate (onychoschizia)
    - ◦ Also, onycholysis, longitudinal striation (onychorrhexis), subungual hyperkeratosis, or anonychia
- Drug-related
    - ◦ β-blockers
    - ◦ Antimalarials
    - ◦ Captopril
    - ◦ Gold
    - ◦ Penicillamine
    - ◦ HCTZ
    - ◦ NSAIDs

Psoriasis

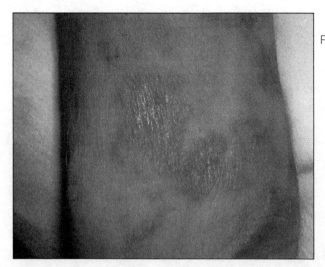

Figure 6.5: Psoriasis

- Affects approximately 2% of population of US
- Usually begins in 3rd decade of life
- An early onset predicts more severe disease
  - Early onset more likely with positive family history

Clinical Manifestations

- Sharply demarcated papules and plaques
- Non-coherent silvery scales
- Auspitz sign → bleeding upon removal of scale
- Koebnerization, stimulation of clinical disease due to external trauma, is seen in 20%
- Woronoff ring: Area of blanching around psoriatic plaques secondary to decrease in prostaglandin, PGE
- Clinical subtypes
  - Guttate

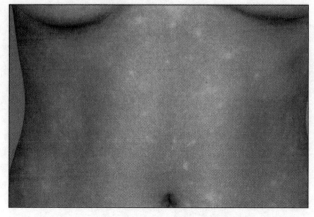

Figure 6.6: Guttate psoriasis

- Small (0.5 to 1.5 cm) lesions over upper trunk and proximal extremities
- Early age of onset/young adults
  - Streptococcal throat infection frequently precedes eruption
  - Generalized pustular
- Fever, lasting several days, with eruption of sterile pustules 2 to 3 mm diameter paralleling the fever

- Fingertips may become anonychia and atrophic
- Hypocalcemia, albuminemia, and leukocytosis
- Can be induced following cessation of systemic steroids
  ○ Psoriatic nail disease

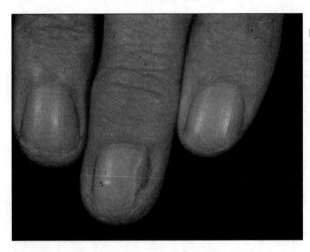

Figure 6.7: Nail psoriasis - Pits and onycholysis

- May be of nail matrix or nail bed origin
- Fingernails involved in 50%, toenails in 35%
- Nail changes more frequent (80 to 90%) in patients with arthritis
- Psoriatic nail changes of matrix → pits (the most common nail change of psoriasis and representing focal psoriasis of the proximal matrix) and leukonychia
  - Pits in psoriasis are generally more randomly distributed than the regular rows of pits seen in alopecia areata
- Psoriatic nail changes of nail bed origin include: Salmon spots, "oil spots," onycholysis, subungual hyperkeratosis, and splinter hemorrhages
- Drugs that exacerbate:
  ○ Steroid withdrawal
  ○ Lithium
  ○ β-blockers
  ○ Interferons
  ○ ACE inhibitors
  ○ G-CSF
- Systemic associations
  ○ Psoriatic arthritis
  ○ Crohn's disease and ulcerative colitis
  ○ HTN, obesity, diabetes, and chronic oropharyngeal infections found more frequently in psoriatic patients
  ○ Increased risk of lymphoma

Treatment
- Topical agent examples:
  ○ Vitamin D3 analogues
    - Calcipotriol, tacalcitol, calcitriol
    - Inhibit keratinocyte proliferation and induce terminal differentiation
    - Anti-inflammatory

- Tazarotene
  - Retinoid
  - Reduces scaling and plaque thickness, with little effectiveness on erythema
- Topical steroids
- Systemic agent examples:
  - Methotrexate
    - Synthetic analog of folic acid that competitively inhibits dihydrofolate reductase
    - Inhibits S phase of cell cycle (like hydroxyurea)
    - Leukopenia and thrombocytopenia indicate overdose → leucovorin rescue required
    - Careful in kidney dysfunction → renal excretion
    - Acute interstitial pneumonitis (rare)
    - Hepatotoxicity; exclude those with liver disease or alcohol abuse
  - Cyclosporine
    - Inhibits release of cytokines, specifically IL-2, by binding and deactivating calcineurin
    - Effective in erythrodermic and generalized pustular psoriasis
    - SE
      - Hypertension (treat with ACE-inhibitors)
      - Elevated triglycerides
      - Hyperkalemia
      - Hypomagnesemia
      - Hepatotoxicity
      - Hypertrichosis (common), gingival hyperplasia, trichomegaly, nausea, vomiting, diarrhea, arthralgia, myalgia, tremor, acne, sebaceous hyperplasia, and fatigue may occur
      - Metabolized by P450, thus erythromycin or ketoconazole will increase drug levels
  - Biologics
    - Biologic therapy refers to proteins synthesized through recombinant DNA techniques as immunomodulating agents
    - Recombinant human cytokines, humanized monoclonal antibodies, or specific molecular receptors
    - Psoriasis is currently the major target for biologic therapies
    - With regard to psoriasis therapy, there are 3 classes of biologics: The T-cell targeting drugs (alefacept), the TNF-inhibiting drugs (etanercept, adalimumab, and infliximab), and newest, il-12/23 (ustekinumab)

Seborrheic Dermatitis
- Related to Malassezia furfur and sebum production
- Seen in infants and post-pubertal
- Face/scalp/chest/back/intertriginous areas
- Salmon colored, waxy scaling patches and plaques
- Severe cases in: HIV, Parkinson's
- Seborrheic dermatitis like: Langerhans cell histiocytosis
- Treatment: Topical steroids, ketoconazole, topical tacrolimus/pimecrolimus

Pityriasis Rosea

Figure 6.8: Herald patch of pityriasis rosea

- Associated with HHV-6 and 7; may be a viral exanthem
- Herald patch (precedes eruption)
- Clears within 6 to 8 weeks
- Tends to be in body folds, e.g., "Christmas tree" distribution
  - Usually spares lower extremities
- Erythromycin can accelerate clearance of PR
- Variant: Inverse PR (involves face, axillae, inguinal areas)
- Always check an RPR in PR (Ddx secondary syphilis)
- PR-like drug eruption: ACEI, gold
- Pityriasis rosea may cause premature delivery with neonatal hypotonia and possibly fetal death especially in the 1st 15 weeks of gestation

Erythema Multiforme

- Target lesion = dusky center, white ring, with surrounding erythema; tend to occur on face, mucosal, acral sites, genitalia
  - Note: Steven Johnson syndrome (SJS) and toxic epidermolytic necrolysis (TEN) are now thought to be variants within a spectrum; erythema multiforme is considered distinct, though with clinical overlap
- Erythema multiforme minor
  - #1 cause = HSV; outbreak precedes EM by 3 to 14 days
  - No systemic or mucosal involvement
- Erythema multiforme major
  - Caused by infection in 90% (HSV, *Mycoplasma*), rarely drugs
  - Has systemic or mucosal involvement
  - Full development of all lesions in 24 to 72 hours, last at least a week
  - Does not progress to TEN
- Rowell syndrome
  - Patients with SLE develop lesions of erythema multiforme

Drug Reactions

- Drug eruptions (adults > children)
- Drug exanthem

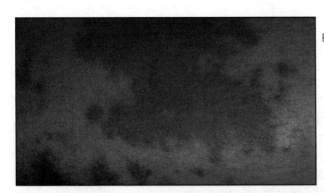

Figure 6.9: Morbilliform drug eruption

- Includes morbilliform drug eruption (i.e., "maculopapular")
- Classically occurs 7 to 14 days after exposure; commonly from PCN/sulfa/anti-convulsant/allopurinol/cephalosporin
- Occurs faster upon re-exposure
- Will occur when PCN (amoxicillin) given for mononucleosis
- Serum-sickness like eruption (fever, arthralgias, urticarial, or morbilliform rash) can occur 1 to 3 weeks; after cefaclor most commonly
- Urticaria/angioedema (discussed in detail below)
  - Most common cause of anaphylaxis: ASA
- Hypersensitivity vasculitis
  - Palpable purpura – non-blanching erythematous papules
  - Papules, urticaria, angioedema, pustules, vesicles, ulcers, necrosis, and livedo reticularis
  - Usually occurs on lower extremities or over dependent areas such as the back and gluteal regions
  - Drug induced:
    - Penicillin
    - Sulfonamides
    - Thiazides
    - Allopurinol
    - Phenytoin
    - NSAIDs
    - PTU and hydralazine in association with ANCA
    - Streptokinase
    - Radiocontrast media
    - Monoclonal antibodies
    - G-CSF
- Erythroderma
  - High BSA with erythema
  - Medical emergency due to inability to thermoregulate
- Stevens-Johnsons syndrome/toxic epidermal necrolysis (SJS/TEN), rarely from EM-Major
  - BSA = % of skin with epidermal detachment (<10% in EM-Major, 10 to 30% in SJS, >30% in TEN)
  - 7 to 21 days after exposure
  - Path: Apoptotic keratinocytes to full epidermal necrosis
  - SJS in 1/106 of general population, 1/1000 of HIV/AIDS (acquired glutathione deficiency)

- Hypersensitivity syndromes
  - Seen most often with anticonvulsants and sulfonamides, and less commonly with allopurinol, dapsone, and gold
    - Reactions present with fever, rash with facial edema, eosinophilia, lymphadenopathy, hepatitis, and nephritis
    - Pathogenesis of anticonvulsant hypersensitivity is related to the individual's inability to detoxify arene oxide metabolites of these medications, due to lack of epoxide hydrolase
      - Diphenylhydantoin, phenobarbital, and carbamazepine are known to cross-react, whereas valproic acid generally does not cross react
- DRESS (Drug reaction with eosinophilia and systemic symptoms)
  - Also known as drug/dilantin hypersensitivity syndrome
  - Most common from aromatic antiepileptic agents
    - Phenytoin, carbamazepine, and phenobarbital (these 3 cross-react) and the sulfonamides, allopurinol
  - Predisposed to by epoxide hydrolase deficiency (anti-epileptics), slow acetylator (sulfas)
  - Can be difficult to distinguish from serum sickness
  - 15 to 40 days after exposure
  - Clinically, facial edema is hallmark
  - Usually see elevation in LFTs (liver most commonly involved)
  - Possible role of HHV-6 and 7 has been proposed
  - Monitor TFTs for 12 weeks; hypothyroidism possible
    - 10% mortality
- Acute generalized exanthematous pustulosis (AGEP)
  - Non-follicular, sterile pustules on erythematous background; ddx pustular psoriasis, candidiasis
  - Caused by beta-lactams, macrolides, terbinafine
  - <4 days after exposure
  - Can be associated with elevated WBC (18 to 25)
  - Patch testing positive in 80%
  - Can see upregulated IL-8 (neutrophil chemoattractant)

Specific Drug Eruptions
- Systemic lupus-like eruption
  - Anticonvulsants
  - Isoniazid
  - Hydralazine
  - Minocycline
  - Procainamide
  - Penicillin
  - D-penicillamine
- Subacute cutaneous lupus-like eruption
  - Azathioprine
  - Glyburide
  - Griseofulvin
  - Terbinafine

- ◦ Hydrochlorothiazide
- ◦ Penicillin
- ◦ Penicillamine
- Acne-inducing drugs
  - ◦ ACTH
  - ◦ Steroids
  - ◦ Halogens
  - ◦ Lithium
  - ◦ INH
  - ◦ Dilantin

6.3 INFLAMMATORY DISEASES OF THE ADNEXA

Acne

Pathogenesis

- Follicular hyperkeratosis
- Microcomedone is precursor lesion
- Human sebum is rich in triglycerides
  - ◦ P. acnes makes an enzymatic lipase which cleaves triglycerides into free fatty acids
- P. acnes can activate complement and PMNs chemotaxis
  - ◦ IL-1 contributes
- Toll-like receptors
  - ◦ Recognize bacterial patterns
  - ◦ P. acnes activates TLR-2
  - ◦ Certain retinoids downregulate TLR-2

Clinical

- Acne vulgaris
  - ◦ Open = "black head" and closed = "white head"
  - ◦ Inflammatory lesions are papules, pustules and nodules

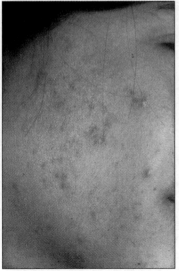

Figure 6.10: Acne vulgaris

- Acne fulminans
  - Explosive: Trunk > face
  - Leukocytosis, fever, arthralgias
  - Lytic bone changes
  - Sternoclavicular joints and chest wall inflammation
  - Tx with prednisone and isotretinoin
- Chloracne
  - Malar, postauricular, scrotum
  - Cutting oils and dioxin
- Acne-like induced eruptions
  - Halogens, bromide, and iodide
  - Androgenetic hormones such as testosterone, ACTH, corticosteroids
  - Isoniazid (INH)
  - Lithium
  - Erbitux
  - Phenytoin
  - Cyclosporine
  - Vitamins B2, B6, and B12

Treatment
- Erythromycin and clindamycin less effective against P. acnes
- Tetracyclines below MIC can inhibit PMNs, cytokines and P. acnes production of lipase
  - Risk of photosensitivity demecycline > doxycycline > tetracycline > minocycline
  - Unlike other tetracyclines, doxycycline is excreted via the GI tract rather than the kidneys, and thus is the tetracycline of choice in renal-compromised patients
  - Minocycline can cause hyperpigmentation of the skin. Three types are generally described:
    - Blue-black discoloration: Appearing in areas of prior skin injury, such as acne scars
    - Blue-gray discoloration: Often at the lower anterior legs and forearms
    - Muddy brown discoloration: Found on sun-exposed areas. The least common type of hyperpigmentation
- Only rifampin reduces OCP efficacy in studies
- Isotretinoin
  - 120-150 mg/kg total dose
  - SE: Pseudotumor with TCN
  - Large study failed to show increased risk of suicide
  - Large study failed to show association with IBD
- Hormonal
  - Estrogen
    - Ethinyl estradiol most common
    - Desogestrel, norgestimate and gestodene lowest andro properties
    - Combo works best
  - Anti-androgen
    - Spironolactone

Rosacea

Clinical

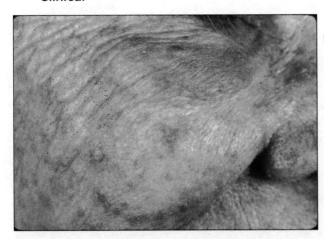

Figure 6.11: Papulopustular rosacea

- Papules and papulopustules in central region of face against a vivid background of telangiectases
  - Later, diffuse hyperplasia of connective tissue with enlarged sebaceous glands
- Localized to nose, cheeks, chin, forehead, glabella; less commonly affected areas include the retroauricular, V-shaped chest area, neck, back, scalp
- Flushing and blushing evoked by UV, heat, cold, chemical irritation, strong emotions, alcoholic beverages, hot drinks, and spices
- Variants of rosacea
  - Persistent edema of rosacea (rosacea lymphedema or Morbihan's disease)
    - Often misdiagnosed as cellulitis
  - Ophthalmic rosacea
    - Blepharitis, conjunctivitis, iritis, keratitis (inflammation of cornea)
    - The treatment of choice for ocular rosacea is oral antibiotics
  - Granulomatous rosacea
    - Dozens of brown-red papules or nodules on diffusely reddened skin, frequently involving lower eyelids
  - Steroid rosacea
    - Steroid atrophy with resultant telangiectases
    - Flaming red, scaling, papule-covered face
    - Withdrawal of steroid accompanied by exacerbation of disease
      - Slow tapering of steroid over months is required
  - Rosacea fulminans (Pyoderma faciale)
    - Occurs almost exclusively in post-adolescent women; lots of flushing and blushing
  - Perioral dermatitis
    - May be triggered or exacerbated by topical steroid use
    - Spares vermillion border
  - Phymas
    - Rhinophyma
      - Occurs almost exclusively in men
    - Gnathophyma: Chin swelling
    - Metophyma: Forehead and nose saddle

- Otophyma: Earlobes
- Blepharophyma: Eyelids

Treatment
- Topical
  - Antibiotics – often effective
    - Topical metronidazole active against papules and pustules, but not telangiectasia and flushing
    - Topical sulfur-based preparations
  - Azelaic acid
  - Sunscreen
- Systemic
  - Antibiotics – generally responds well – Tetracyclines
  - Isotretinoin – indicated in phymas; but rosacea often rapidly recurs after discontinuation of isotretinoin

Hidradenitis Suppurativa
- Component of follicular occlusion triad
  - Acne conglobata, hidradenitis suppurativa, and dissecting cellulitis of the scalp
- Associated with smoking and being overweight
- Hidradenitis suppurativa severity predictors
  - Atypical locations more common in men than in women
    - Men have more severe disease
  - Increased body mass index
  - Atypical locations
  - A personal history of severe acne
    - Absence of a family history of HS were associated with more severe disease
- Clinical: Recurrent, inflamed cystic nodules in intertriginous areas. Chronic inflammation can lead to the formation of sinus tracts
- Treatment: Topical antibiotics (i.e., clindamycin), antibacterial washes, oral antibiotics (rifampin + clindamycin > tetracycline class), oral retinoids

6.4 FUNGAL SKIN AND NAIL INFECTIONS

Superficial Fungal Infections

Tinea Versicolor
- Malassezia globosa #1 cause – Lipophilic
- Clinical: White or brown flat, small scaly plaques in seborrheic distribution (usually spares face)
- Wood's lamp yellow
- Tx: Topical antifungals and selenium sulfide-containing shampoos

Tinea Nigra
- Phaeoannellomyces werneckii
- Palms, soles
- Dark organisms in stratum corneum

Dermatophytosis

- Dermatophytes: Group of closely related filamentous fungi, which colonize keratin such as the stratum corneum of the epidermis, hair, nails, feathers of various animals
    - 3 subtypes: Microsporum, Epidermophyton (never impacts hair bearing areas), and Trichophyton
- T. capitis – Dermatophyte infection of the scalp and hair, generally seen in childhood
    - Significant posterior cervical lymphadenopathy is noted
    - Ectothrix
        - Fluorescent (mostly microsporum)
        - Non-fluorescent (mostly trichophyton)
    - Endothrix = Black dot ringworm – invades the hair shaft so breaks
    - Favus = Scutula - yellowish cups with hair penetrating though
        - T. schoenleinii, violaceum, gypseum
    - Kerion
        - Boggy, oozing inflammatory reaction to fungus
        - Regional lymphadenopathy
        - Scarring alopecia may result
        - May need prednisone
- T. corporis

Figure 6.12: Tinea corporis

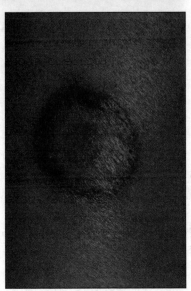

Figure 6.13: Tinea corporis

- Organisms invade stratum corneum generally causing an annular lesion with an erythematous raised, scaly advancing border, the center of the lesion may show clearing

- Majocchi's granuloma
  - Indurated, pink plaque with prominent hair follicles caused by T. rubrum
  - Needs systemic antifungals
- T. barbae
  - In men, the bearded area of the face and neck, generally inflammatory
  - Associated with exposure to animals
- T. cruris
  - Mainly seen in males, involves the groin, perineal and perianal skin
  - Direct or indirect contact
- T. pedis - 3 clinical subtypes:
  - Moccasin
  - Interdigital
  - Bullous
  - Interweb infections often involve fungi, yeast, gram negative and positive bacteria
- Onychomycosis
  - Fungal infection of the nails due to dermatophyte, yeast, or nondermatophyte
  - Clinical subtypes
    - Distal lateral subungual onychomycosis
      - Infection begins distally and involves the nail bed, nail plate and lateral nail fold; thick nail with debris, loose or cracked nail plate
    - Proximal white subungual onychomycosis
      - Rarest form of onychomycosis
      - AIDS marker
      - Organisms enter the cuticle and infect the proximal part of the nail bed causing white islands that slowly invade the nail plate
    - White Superficial Onychomycosis
      - Organism invades the surface of the nail plate of toenails only
      - Irregular white chalky opaque patches on the nail

Candidiasis
- Candida albicans, C. glabrata (fluconazole resistant), C. parapsilosis, C. tropicalis, C. krusei, C. dubliniensis (thrush in HIV)
- Most common fungal opportunistic infection, may be difficult to evaluate; yeast are ubiquitous and part of endogenous flora
- Prototypically bright red, moist patches with satellite pustules
- Intertriginous involvement or thrush
- Factors contributing to candida infection:
  - Impaired epithelial cell barrier, systemic illness, neutrophil and macrophage disorders, immune disorders, therapeutic agents, congenital or acquired endocrine disorders, malignancies, indwelling catheters, hyperalimentation, heat, humidity, and friction
- Clinical variants
  - Angular cheilitis: A classic complication of childhood diabetes, presents as a white curd-like material adherent to red, fissured oral commissures
  - Median rhomboid glossitis
  - Chronic paronychia: Involves the proximal nailfold; erythema, swelling, separation from the nail margin with nail dystrophy
    - C. parapsilosis

- Super infection by bacterial organisms, most commonly S. aureus, may occur causing an acute paronychia
  ○ Erosio interdigitalis blastomycetica: Interdigital infection between the 3rd and 4th fingers or 4th and 5th toes

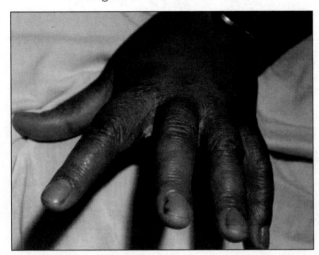

Figure 6.14: Erosio interdigitalis blastomycetica

  ○ Genital infections: Vulvovaginitis and candida intertrigo of the inframammary region in women
    - In contrast, balanitis and phimosis in men are relatively less common
- Treatment includes control of blood sugar and topical or systemic antifungals

6.5 BACTERIAL INFECTIONS

Anthrax

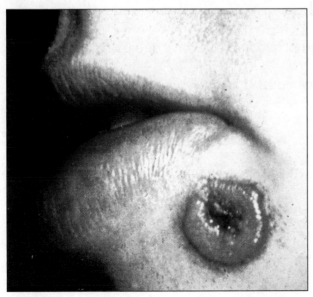

Figure 6.15: Malignant pustule of anthrax

- Bacillus anthracis – Spore-forming, gram+ rod
- Animal exposure
- Exotoxins
  - Edema toxin = Edema factor (EF) + protective antigen (PA)
    - EF causes gelatinous edema by increasing camp
  - Lethal toxin = Lethal factor (LF) + PA
    - LF can cause shock and death in disseminated disease by release of TNF and IL-1 – PA allows entry of exotoxins into the cells
    - Antibodies to PA will prevent LF and EF action
- 3 clinical forms:
  - Inhalational, GI, and cutaneous
  - Cutaneous
    - Malignant pustule followed by bullae and eschar
- Treatment
  - Conventional—PCN
  - Bioterrorism—ciprofloxacin or doxycycline

Borrelia
- Lyme
  - Tick-borne
    - Organism: B. burgdorferi
    - Vector: Ixodes dammini, pacificus, ricinus

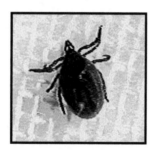 Figure 6.16: Ixodes

  - Clinical: Erythema migrans, chronica atrophicans (rare, chronic disease resulting in acral sclerodermoid changes
  - Treatment: Doxycycline – Amoxicillin for kids and pregnant women
- Relapsing fever
  - Louse-borne
    - Organism: B. recurrentis
    - Vector: Pediculus humulus
  - Clinical fever, HA, systemic disease
  - Treatment: Doxycycline
- Relapsing fever
  - Tick-borne
    - Organism: B. duttonii
    - Vector: Ornithodoros soft tick
  - Same symptoms as above
  - Treatment: Doxycycline

Botryomycosis
- Staph, E. coli, pseudomonas, and proteus
- Granulomatous nodules or plaques
- Clinical setting: Immunosuppression

Staphylococcus aureus
- Toxic shock syndrome
  - Enterotoxins B and C
  - TSST-1 in menstrual cases
  - Scarlatiniform eruption and desquamation with <u>sepsis</u>
- Staph scalded skin syndrome
  - Exfoliative toxin A and B
  - Bind to Desmoglein-1 (a transmembrane adhesion molecule in the epidermis)
  - At risk populations: Kids and renal disease patients
  - Nikolsky sign + in non-lesional skin
  - Culture of bullae useless – no organism present (toxin mediated)
- Bullous impetigo
  - Exfoliative toxin A and B
- Others: Sycosis barbae, Botryomycosis, Acute paronychia, Felon, Endocarditis

Strep spp.
- Group A Strep
  - Blistering distal dactylitis
    - Dorsal fingers and toes
    - Tense blisters
  - Perianal strep
    - <u>Bright</u> red and well-demarcated
  - Scarlet fever
    - Erythrogenic toxin A, B, and C
    - Strep throat
    - Exudative pharyngitis and strawberry tongue
    - Sandpaper rash starts on head and neck
    - Pastia's lines
      - Linear petechiae in axillae and antecubital fossae
  - Purpura fulminans
    - Hemorrhagic infarction from DIC
    - Geographic areas of purpura
  - Others: Non-bullous impetigo, erysipelas, cellulitis (see Figure), necrotizing fasciitis, Strep toxic-shock-like syndrome, endocarditis

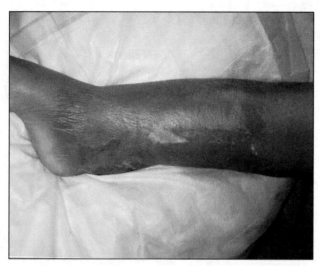

Figure 6.17: Cellulitis

Meningococcemia

- N. meningitides
  - ◦ Gram negative diplococcus
- Those at risk: Children and those with complement deficiencies (C3-5)
- Petechiae may be 1st sign
- IV PCN or ceftriaxone

Rhinoscleroma

- Klebsiella pneumoniae rhinoscleromatis
- Plaques on external nares
- Mikulicz cells on path
- Tx: Cipro

Pseudomonal Skin Infections

- Ecthyma gangrenosum
  - ◦ *P. aeruginosa* (PA)
  - ◦ At risk: Immunocompromised patients
  - ◦ Starts as hemorrhagic vesicle, pustule, and develops to necrosis
    - Assume sepsis
- Green nails
  - ◦ PA
  - ◦ Pyocyanin – virulence factor/cause of color
- Gram negative toe web infection
  - ◦ PA, E. coli, proteus
  - ◦ Typically starts with dermatophytosis
- Blastomycosis-like pyoderma
  - ◦ PA and S. aureus
- Hot tub folliculitis
  - ◦ PA
  - ◦ Self-limiting – 1 to 4 days after soaking
  - ◦ Rarely patients get malignant otitis from PA

Rickettsial

Table 6.2: Rickettsial Diseases

	Causative Organism	Vector
Rocky Mountain spotted fever	*R. rickettsii*	1.) Western US - *Dermacentor andersoni* 2.) Eastern US - *Dermacentor variabilis*
Rickettsialpox	*R. akari*	*Liponyssoides sanguineus* - Mite of the house mouse
Epidemic typhus	*R. prowazekii*	*Pediculus humanus corporis* - human body louse
Endemic typhus	*R. typhi*	*Xenopsylla cheopis* - rat flea
Scrub fyphus	*Orientia tsutsugamushi*	Chiggers - trombiculid mite larvae
Q Fever	*Coxiella burnetii*	Dried tick feces which are inhaled
Ehrlichiosis 1.) Human monocytic ehrlichiosis 2.) Human granulocytic ehrlichiosis	1.) *E. chaffeensis* 2.) Human Granylocytic Ehrlichiosis (HGE) agent	1.) *Amblyomma anericanum* 2.) *Ixodes sapularis, Ixodes pacificus*

- Caused by obligate intracellular coccobacilli
- Transmitted by arthropod vectors
- Tx: Tetracyclines (doxycycline preferred)

Mycobacterial

- Leprosy

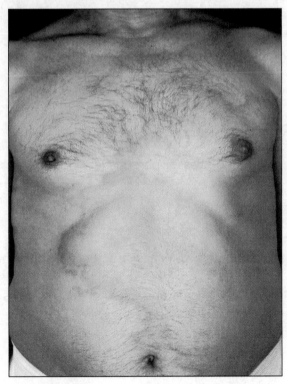

Figure 6.18: Leprosy

Table 6.3: Leprosy

TT	BT	BB	BL	LL
TH1 cytokine profile: IFN-γ, IL-2, IL-12 Paucibacillary Lepromin test+	⟵		⟶	TH2 cytokine profile IL-4, IL-10 Multibacillary Lepromin test-
≤3 lesions	3–10 lesions that are smaller than TT lesions	Many lesions distributed asymmetrically	Lesions too numerous to count; smaller predominate	Generalized and symmetrical distribution
Anesthetic and anhidrotic lesions	Similar to TT	Less anesthesia than TT	Minimal or no sensory defects	No loss of sensation or sweating

Table 6.4: Treatment (WHO Recommendations)

Paucibacillary	Dapsone 100 mg po qd for 6 months Rifampin 600 mg po q monthly for 6 months
Multibacillary	Dapsone 100 mg po qd for 12 months Clofazimine 50 mg po qd for 12 months Rifampin 600 mg po q monthly for 12 months Clofazimine 300 mg po q monthly for 12 months (supervised)

- ○ Causative organism: Mycobacterium leprae
  - Transmitted from human to human most likely via respiratory secretions
  - Spectrum of disease based on cell mediated immune response
  - Armadillos may be a nonhuman source of infection
- Miliary tuberculosis of the skin
  - ○ Hematogenous spread of mycobacteria from fulminant tuberculosis of the lung or meninges
    - Immunosuppressed host HIV, infants
    - Tuberculin test is negative (anergic)
  - ○ Disseminated erythematous macules, papules, nodules, or purpuric lesions
- Atypical mycobacteria
  - ○ M. fortuitum, M. chelonei, M. abscessus
    - "Rapid growers"
    - Found in soil, water, dust, and animals
    - Infections occur after exposure to contaminated surgical instruments or following trauma
    - Typically presents with a single or multiple erythematous subcutaneous nodules on an extremity
    - Treatment: Surgical drainage/debridement followed by course of antimicrobial therapy (amikacin, clarithromycin, ciprofloxacin, imipenem, and others)
  - ○ M. Marinum
    - Swimming pool/aquarium granuloma
    - Begins as small papule at site of inoculation and evolves into a nodule or granulomatous plaque, often with a verrucous surface
    - Treatment: Minocycline

Table 6.5: Tuberculosis of the Skin (Summary)

Tuberculous Chancre	Tuberculosis Verrucosa Cutis	Lupus Vulgaris	Scrofuloderma	Tuberculous Gumma	Tuberculosis Cutis Orificialis
Primary (exogenous) inoculation	Exogenous re-infection	Hematogenous, lymphatic, or contiguous spread from distant site of tuberculous infection	Contiguous spread onto skin from underlying tuberculous infection	Hematogenous spread	Autoinoculation from underlying advanced visceral tuberculosis
Non-sensitized host	Sensitzed host with strong immunity	Sensitized host with moderate to high immunity	Sensitized host with low immunity	Immuno-suppressed host	Sensitized host with diminishing immunity
Pauci- or Multi-bacillary, depending on stage of infection and strength of immune response	Paucibacillary	Pauci-bacillary	Multi- or pauci-bacillary	Multi-bacillary	Multi-bacillary
· Painless red-brown papule that ulcerates · Tuberculous primary complex: regional hadenopathy, 3-8 weeks post infection	· Slowly growing verrucous plaques with irregular borders · Typically on hand	· Brownish-red plaque · "Apple-jelly" color on diascopy · Head/neck involvement in 90% of cases	· Subcutaneous nodules with purulent or caseous drainage · May develop sinuses and ulcers with granulating bases · Occurs most commonly over cervical lymph nodes	· Subcutaneous abscesses · May form fistulas and ulcers · Typically on trunk, head, or extremities	· Punched-out ulcers with undermined edges · On ucocutaneous junctions of mouth, genitalia

6.6 VIRAL INFECTIONS

DNA Viruses

- CMV
  - Infection during 1st and 2nd trimester - highest risk for permanent abnormalities
    - Small for gestational age, microcephaly, retinitis, colobomas, intracranial calcifications
    - #1 infectious cause of deafness and mental retardation in US
    - Most common congenital viral infection
    - Part of TORCH syndrome – with "blueberry muffin baby" purpura
- EBV
  - Infects B lymphocytes
  - Infectious mononucleosis

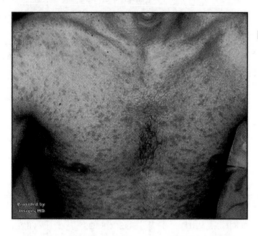

Figure 6.19: Mononucleosis

  - Fever, pharyngitis, and lymphadenopathy
  - Malaise, headache, myalgias, hepatosplenomegaly
  - Commonly morbilliform eruption after treatment with ampicillin
  - Affects teenagers and young adults
  - Oral hairy leukoplakia
    - Raised white plaque on lateral tongue
    - HIV and other immunocompromised states
- Exanthem subitum
  - HHV 6,7
  - High fever followed by pink macules and papules – resolves with fever (1 to 2 days)
  - Starts on trunk

Human Papillomavirus (HPV)

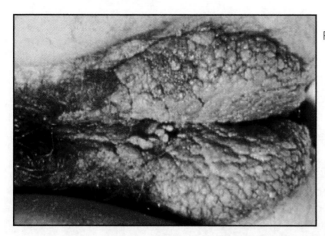

Figure 6.20: Condyloma

- Genome encodes "E" (early) and "L" (late proteins)
  - E proteins (E1-8): Participate in viral DNA replication
  - L proteins (L1-L2): Structural proteins – form virion (the outer shell of the virus)

Herpes Simplex Virus (HSV-1, HSV-2)

Clinical Presentations

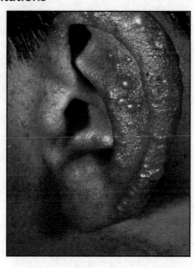

Figure 6.21: Herpes simplex 1

- Primary gingivostomatitis
  - Seen in children and young adults following primary HSV infection (usually HSV-1); occurs in only 1% of primary HSV infections of the lips or face
  - Presents with fever, sore throat, and painful vesicles/erosions on the tongue, palate, buccal, and gingival mucosa
  - Erosions are covered with characteristic gray membrane
- Primary genital herpes
  - Most cases caused by primary infection with HSV-2
  - Multiple painful erosions, often bilateral, on the ano-genital mucosa
  - Painful inguinal lymphadenopathy

- Minority of cases may have concomitant aseptic meningitis with fever, nuchal rigidity, headache, photophobia
  - Dysuria and vaginal/urethral discharge may be present
  - Severity of symptoms peaks at days 8 to 10
- Herpes gladiatorum
  - Affects wrestlers and rugby players
  - Most common locations: Face, lateral neck, medial arm
- Neonatal herpes simplex
  - Majority of cases acquired during delivery as neonate passes through infected vaginal canal
  - Clinical spectrum ranges from localized skin lesions to multi-systemic infection with encephalitis, hepatitis, pneumonia, and coagulopathy
- Herpes simplex treatment
  - Acyclovir
    - Guanosine analogue
    - Inhibits viral DNA polymerase after being phosphorylated by viral thymidine kinase (TK), and 2 additional viral kinases
  - Famciclovir
    - Prodrug of penciclovir; Increased bioavailability and longer half-life
    - Also dependent on viral TK for activity
  - Valacyclovir
    - Viral TK-dependent; same mechanism of action as acyclovir
    - Thrombotic thrombocytopenic purpura reported using high doses in immunosuppressed patients
  - Acyclovir-resistant HSV* – treatment
    - *Most commonly due to TK-deficient strains of HSV
    - Foscarnet – directly inhibits viral DNA polymerase (without requiring phosphorylation by TK)
    - Cidofovir – inhibits viral DNA polymerase in a TK-independent fashion

Varicella (Varicella-Zoster Virus)

- Distinguishing features (compared to smallpox):
  - Absent or mild prodrome
  - Lesions begin on face and spread to trunk
  - Centripetal distribution with fewest lesions on extremities
  - "Dew drops on a rose petal" – superficial vesicle with erythematous halo
  - Lesions in different stages of evolution
  - Rapid evolution (<24 h) of lesions from macule-papule-vesicle-crust
  - Varicella in pregnancy
    - 1st 20 weeks of gestation: Congenital varicella syndrome - hypoplastic limbs, ocular and CNS abnormalities
    - 5 days before and 2 days after delivery: Neonatal varicella
      - Neonate develops varicella at 5 to 10 days of age because of inadequate transplacental delivery of maternal anti-varicella antibodies
      - Treat with VZIG + IV-acyclovir

Herpes Zoster (Varicella-Zoster Virus)

- ∘ Ramsay Hunt syndrome
  - Caused by VZV infection of the geniculate ganglion
  - Zoster involves the external ear
  - Facial paralysis – ipsilateral
  - Tinnitus or other auditory symptom

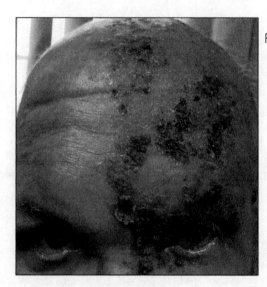

Figure 6.22: Herpes zoster

Other Human Herpes Viruses

- HHV-6: Causes roseola infantum = exanthem subitum = Sixth disease
- HHV-7: Also causes roseola
- HHV-8: Oncogenic virus: Kaposi's sarcoma, Castleman syndrome

Milker's Nodule

- Paravaccinia virus
- Cows
- 1 cm nodule on arm or finger
- No treatment necessary

Molluscum

- Poxvirus
- Clinical: Umbilicated white papules

Orf

- Parapoxvirus
- Sheep and goats
- Dorsal index finger
- 6 stages: Papular, target, acute, regenerative, papillomatous, regressive

Parvovirus B19 (the only ssDNA virus)

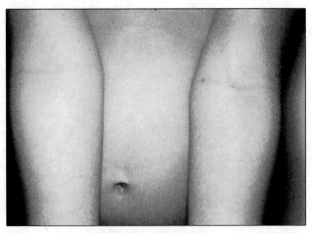

Figure 6.23: Reticulated erythema of Fifth disease

- Erythema infectiosum or fifth disease
- Clinical: Children - slapped cheek erythema progressing to lacy reticular truncal erythema (no longer infectious at this point)
  - <u>Arthropathy</u> in adult
  - Hydrops and spontaneous abortion
  - Purpuric gloves and stocking syndrome
  - Aplastic crisis in sickle cell patients

Smallpox

- Poxvirus - Variola
- Incubation is an average of 12 days
  - Virus replicates during this time
    - Not contagious
  - Prodrome -3 days of fever, malaise, HA, back pain, and vomiting
- Rare swimming trunk petechiae is pathognomonic
- Generalized centrifugal eruption
  - Over 2 weeks
  - Lesions in same stage
  - Umbilicated lesion
  - Head and extremities > trunk
- Most infectious during the 1st 7 to 10 days following rash onset
- Contagious until scabs fall off

RNA Viruses

- Measles
  - Paramyxovirus
    - Clinical
      - Prodrome fever, cough, coryza, and conjunctivitis
      - Enanthem: Koplik spots
      - Exanthem: Morbilliform eruption starting on face
- Hand-foot-and-mouth disease
  - Coxsackievirus A16 or enterovirus 71
  - Oral-oral and fecal-oral mode of transmission

- Erythematous papules with grayish vesicle and surrounding red areola are characteristic cutaneous lesions
- Herpangina
  - Group A coxsackievirus
  - Fever, headache, cervical lymphadenopathy
  - Gray-white papulovesicles in oral mucosa that ulcerate (commonly present on tonsillar fauces, palate)

Table 6.6 RNA Viruses

Virus Group	Major Examples
Paramyxovirus	Measles, mumps
Togavirus	Rubella
Rhabdovirus	Rabies
Retrovirus	HIV, HTLV
Picornavirus	Enterovirus: Coxsackie virus (Hand-foot-and-mouth disease)

6.7 STDS

	Primary Syphilis	Chancroid	Granuloma Inguinale	Lymphogranuloma Venereum
Causative Organism	*T. pallidum*	*H. ducreyi*	*Calymmatobacterium granulomatis*	*Chlamydia trachomatis L1, L2, L3*
Characteristic Clinical Features	Painless chancre with "ham-colored" base and sharply defined, indurated border Chancre has cartilage-like consistency and exudes clear fluid Bilateral	Soft, painful/tender chancre with ragged edges "School of fish" on Gram or Giemsa stain	Primary lesion: Papule, subcutaneous nodule (pseudobubo), or ulcer 4 clinical forms: Ulcerovegetative (most common), nodular, hypertrophic, and cicatricial Donnovan bodies ("safety-pin" shaped intracytoplasmic inclusions in macrophages) seen on microscopy	Painless, soft erosion that heals spontaneously Secondary inguinal adenopathy with fluctuant, tender nodes above and below Poupart's ligament—"groove sign" (can be bilateral) Serologic diagnosis by complement fixation test
Treatment	Penicillin	Azithromycin Ceftriaxone Ciprofloxacin Erythromycin	TMP-SMX Doxycycline Erythromycin Ciprofloxacin	Doxycycline

Chancroid

- H. ducreyi
- Gram negative rod - "School of fish" appearance
- Painful ulcer
- Tx: Azithromycin

Lymphogranuloma Venereum

- Chlamydia trachomatis L1, 2, 3
- Painless erosion that heals spontaneously
- Fluctuant inguinal lymphadenopathy
  - Groove sign
- Dx: Complement fixation test
- Tx: Doxycycline x 3 weeks

Granuloma Inguinale – Klebsiella Granulomatis (Formerly Calymmatobacterium Granulomatis)

- Gram negative rod
- Safety pin appearance (intracytoplasmic inclusions in macrophages)
- Treatment with sulfamethoxazole and trimethoprim or doxycycline for 3 weeks

Gonococcemia

- N. gonorrhoeae
- Hemorrhagic pustules on red bases
- Arthralgias
- May have C5-C9 deficiency
- Treatment with ceftriaxone

Syphilis

- T. pallidum
- Primary

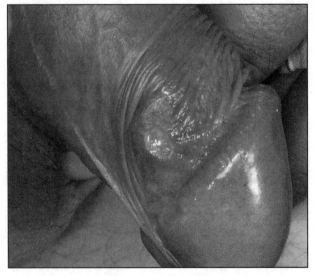

Figure 6.24: Painless chancre of primary syphilis

  - Chancre – 10 days to 3 months after exposure
    - Lasts 3 to 12 weeks

- Secondary

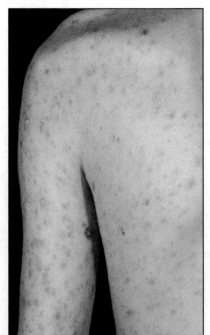

Figure 6.25: Secondary syphilis

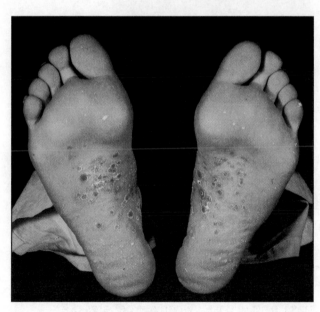

Figure 6.26: Secondary syphilis

  - 4 to 12 weeks
  - Skin and mucous membranes - pityriasis rosea-like
  - Ham-colored macules on palms
  - Condyloma lata
  - Split papules - oral commissures
  - "Moth-eaten" alopecia
- Tertiary
  - Cardiovascular and neurological sequelae in some

- Congenital ~ Secondary syphilis
  - Early <2 years
    - SGA
    - "Saw-tooth" metaphysis
    - "Snuffles
      - Rhinitis
    - Rhagades
    - Parrot's lines
  - Late >2 years (think bony abnormalities)
    - Mulberry molars
    - High-arched palate
    - Hutchinson's teeth (wide spaces and peg-shaped)
    - Saddle nose
    - Saber shins
    - Clutton's joints (non-tender edema of knees)
    - Higoumenakis sign (UL medial clavicle enlargement)
    - Hutchinson's triad – Hutchinson's teeth – deafness – interstitial keratitis

Serology

- Nontreponemal tests
  - VDRL: 4 to 5 weeks after inoculation
    - May revert in latency
  - RPR: Similar to VDRL
- Treponemal
  - FTA-ABS: 3 weeks after inoculation
    - Remains + after treatment
    - Most sensitive test
  - MHA-TP
    - Similar to FTA-ABS, but less sensitive
- Treatment
  - Primary and secondary without end-organ damage
    - Benzathine PCN G 2.4 mil U IM X 1 – doxycycline 100 mg BID x 2 week if PCN allergic
  - Tertiary without neuro disease—benzathine PCN G 2.4 mil U IM weekly X 3
- Jarisch-Herxheimer reaction
  - Fever, HA, LAD, skin lesions, myalgias, WBCs –
  - Caused by TNF-alpha and other cytokines being released when spirochetes are phagocytosed

6.8 PARASITES

Leishmaniasis

- Old World—L. major, tropica, aethiopica, infantum, donovani
- New World—L. mexicana, braziliensis, amazonensis
- Mucocutaneous

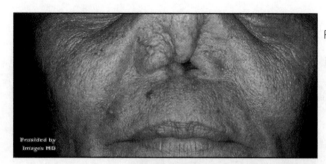

Figure 6.27: Leishmaniasis

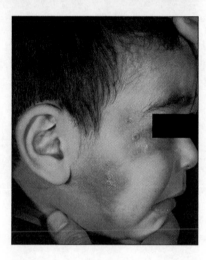

Figure 6.28: Leishmaniasis

- Old World—L. aethiopica
- New World—L. braziliensis
- Visceral
  - L. donovani
  - L. infantum
- Vector
  - Sandflies
    - Old World—Phlebotomus
    - New World—Lutzomyia
- Diagnosis
  - Culture in Novy-MacNeal-Nicolle (NNN) medium
  - Histology
    - Amastigotes in histiocyte cytoplasm
      - Giemsa stain - Kinetoplast
- Treatment
  - Pentavalent antimony/sodium stibogluconate
  - Monitor for cardiac side effects

Trypanosomiasis
- African
  - T. brucei gambiense in West Africa
  - T. brucei rhodesiense in East Africa
  - Vector: Tsetse fly/Glossina
  - Winterbottom's sign
    - Posterior cervical LAD
- American (Chagas disease)
  - T. cruzi
  - Vector: Reduviid beetle aka assassin bug
  - Clinical: Romana sign
    - Eyelid edema and conjunctivitis at site of inoculation
  - Chronic: Cardiac infiltration
  - GI: Toxic megacolon

Filariasis
- Lymphedema and elephantiasis
- Brugia malayi and timori; Wuchereia bancrofti
- Vectors: Mosquitos - Aedes, anopheles, culex, and mansonia

Dracunculiasis
- D. medinensis – Cyclops copepods
- Worms under the skin
- Tx: Slowly remove parasite

Loa Loa
- Mango or deer flies
- Vector: Chrysops
- Clinical: Calabar swellings = dead filarial in microvasculature causing nonpitting edema of cheeks
- "Eye worm"
- Treatment with diethylcarbamazine

Onchocerciasis
- O. volvulus
- Vector: Black flies aka Simulium
- Pruritic papules
- Chronic: Leopard skin, onchocercoma (nodules of organism)
- River Blindness: # 1 cause of acquired blindness worldwide
- Treatment with ivermectin
- Mazzotti reaction: Symptom complex seen in patients after undergoing treatment of onchocerciasis with the medication diethylcarbamazine (DEC)
  - Life-threatening, and are characterized by fever, urticaria, swollen and tender lymph nodes, tachycardia, hypotension, arthralgias, oedema, and abdominal pain

Strongyloidiasis
- S. stercoralis
- Larvae penetrates through skin or mucous membrane

- Clinical entity - Larva currens (STRONG CURRENt)
- Serpiginous urticarial plaques on lower extremities
- Disseminated - thumbprint purpura on periumbilical skin along with petechiae

Cercarial Dermatitis
- "Swimmer's itch"
- Penetrate skin while swimming in northern US or Canadian waters
- Pruritic papules on non-covered skin

Seabather's Eruption
- Edwardsiella lineata—sea anemone
- Linuche unguiculata—thimble jellyfish
- Eruption is on covered skin - pressure from clothing releases toxin

6.9 BITES AND STINGS

Overview
- Eruptions are caused by venom, bites, allergic/irritant response, or systemic reactions
  - Mites, spiders, ticks, and scorpions = arachnids (8 legs)
  - Lice and bees/wasps = insects (6 legs)

Mites
- Scabies

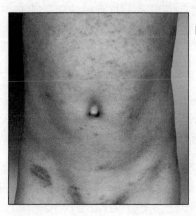

Figure 6.29: Scabies

  - Extremely pruritic burrows/papules in skin folds and acral webs, transmitted through physical contact, particularly in crowded jails, college housing, and nursing homes
  - Can have atypical presentation in infants – bullous, involve the genitals
  - Testing = scabies prep skin scraping showing scabies mites, eggs, or feces
  - Treatment = permethrin 5% cream repeated in 7 days, severe cases oral ivermectin, linens/clothing washed in hot water

Ticks
- Lyme disease
  - Transmitted by deer ticks, most common vector-borne disease in the US
  - Clinical
    - Early localized = erythema migrans (expanding targetoid rash) 1 to 2 weeks after bite

- Early disseminated = within 6 months of bite, disseminated rash, polyarthritis, Bells palsy
- Late/chronic = months to years later, neurologic and rheumatologic symptoms
  - Serologic testing = unhelpful acutely
  - Treatment = single dosage doxycycline if within 72 hours of confirmed bite to prevent Lyme, otherwise doxycycline (amoxicillin if allergic) x 10 to 14 days
- Rocky Mountain Spotted Fever
  - Transmitted by dog/wood ticks, most common fatal tick-borne illness in US
  - Clinical
    - Acral petechial rash spreading centrally within a week of bite, fever, and headache may precede
    - Serologic testing = unreliable
    - Treatment: Doxycycline x 7 to 14 days (chloramphenicol if severely allergic), delayed treatment leads to hospitalization, death in up to 5% of cases (vascular damage, shock)

Spiders

- Black widow

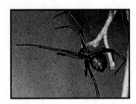

Figure 6.30: Black widow spider

  - Painful edematous bite without necrosis, caused by a neurotoxin mimicking acute abdomen
  - Treatment: Supportive therapy, specific IV antivenin (effective within 4 days of bite), rarely fatal
- Brown recluse
  - Usually painless bite with necrotic skin lesion (erythema/ischemia/thrombosis = red/white/blue), flu-like symptoms, hemolytic anemia, and possible shock/death
  - Treatment: Ice and supportive measures, specific anti-venoms not available

Lice

- Transmitted through physical contact, extreme pruritus and localized lymphadenopathy
  - **Head lice** – Most common louse, laying eggs at the base of hair (nits)
  - **Pubic (crab) lice** – Different body type than other lice (crab-like); macula cerulea = bluish macules in groin (characteristic)
  - **Human body lice** – Located on clothing, not body. Vector for trench fever, epidemic typhus, and relapsing fever
- Treatment: Comb removal of lice/nits, topical permethrin or malathion (flammable) all repeated twice within a week, discarding or laundering clothing/linens in hot water

6.10 COMMON NEOPLASMS

Premalignant and Malignant Tumors

- Typically in sun exposed/sun damaged skin as a new or evolving skin lesion (change of color, size, shape, or new bleeding or irritation)
- Actinic keratosis
  - Keratotic sandpaper-like papules commonly on face and upper extremities, often treated with cryotherapy with liquid nitrogen
- Basal cell carcinoma
  - Pearly telangiectatic pink papules, nodules, patches/plaques; often with rolled border, rarely invasive

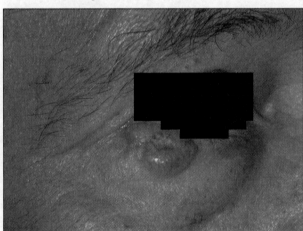

Figure 6.31: Basal cell carcinoma

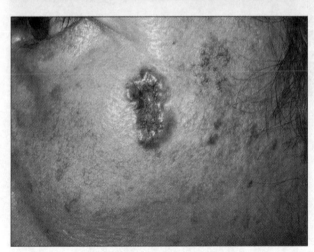

Figure 6.32: Pigmented basal cell carcinoma

- Squamous cell carcinoma
  - Keratotic papules, nodules, patches/plaques; higher risk of invasion if scalp/face

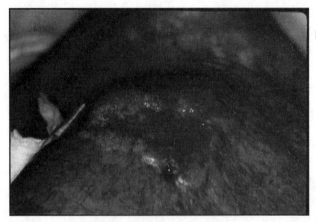

Figure 6.33: Squamous cell carcinoma

  - Nonmelanoma skin cancer treatment = electrodesiccation and curettage, simple excision, or Mohs surgery depending on tumor site and subtype, level of invasion, and size of lesion
- Melanoma

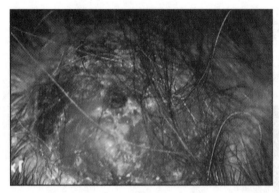

Figure 6.34: Nodular melanoma

  - Brown to black (but can be any color) macule, papule, or nodule with differing clinical features than patient's other skin lesions/nevi, local and distant metastatic potential, can occur anywhere on skin/mucosa
  - **A**(symmetry), **B**(order), **C**(olor), **D**(iameter), **E**(volving)
  - Complete excisional biopsy required for tumor depth (Breslow, determines prognosis)
  - Treatment: Wide local excision, possible sentinel lymph node sampling and body imaging, adjuvant therapies inconsistently effective for metastatic disease, but targeted biologic agents evolving
  - Risk factors for the development of MM include sun exposure with tendency to freckle and sunburn, fair skin complexion, light colored eyes and hair, presence of large number of nevi, as well as family and personal history of melanoma
  - The most important mutated gene associated with a predisposition to develop MM is the CDKN2A (located on chromosome 9p21)

Sun Protection and Skin Cancer Prevention

- Risks of skin cancer
  - Number of blistering sunburns and cumulative exposure to UV light
  - Fairer skin type, genetic factors
  - Geographic locale tanning bed use (artificial UVA/some UVB light)
- Skin cancer prevention/sun protection
  - Seeking shade, particularly 10 am to 2 pm hours when UV light most potent
  - Sun protective clothing, labeled with UPF (ultraviolet protection factor)
  - Sunscreen of SPF (sun protection factor, against UVB rays) >30, with added "broad spectrum" (against UVA rays) and "water resistant" labeling, applied before sun exposure and reapplied at least every 2 hours
  - Avoidance of tanning bed use except if prescribed by a doctor for inflammatory skin disease or part of psychiatric therapy
  - Nightly topical retinoid

6.11 BENIGN TUMORS

- Nevus: Tan to brown papules with genetic and/or environmental triggers, any part of the body
- Seborrheic keratosis: Waxy tan to brown mammillated papules and plaques, often involving the trunk, increasing in number over time particularly in susceptible families

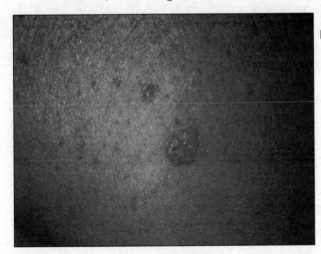

Figure 6.35: Seborrheic keratosis

- Skin tag (acrochordon): Fibrous growth of skin, often multiple tan pedunculated papules particularly in areas of friction, with genetic and metabolic syndrome link
- Corn (clavus): Keratotic firm inverted growth, often on plantar surface, due to friction or pressure
- Epidermoid and pilar cyst: Epidermoid cysts are nodules often with central punctum often on trunk; pilar cysts are dermal nodules with no punctum commonly on the scalp; all have potential for growth and rupture
- Neurofibroma: Pink fleshy papules, sometimes tender; multiple in neurofibromatosis syndromes

- Pyogenic granuloma: Enlarging, easily traumatized red friable papules, can favor the face and digits, more common in children, pregnancy, and with certain HIV drugs; self-resolving but often removed because of tenderness (particularly periungual), and bleeding
- Venous lake: Dark red to purple papule made of blood vessels, commonly on the lip
- Cherry angioma: Red papules favoring the trunk, typically increasing in number over time
- Dermatofibroma: Firm dusky pink to brown papules with "dimple sign" on exam, commonly on legs of females, sometimes precipitated by trauma
- Hypertrophic scars and keloids: Hypertrophic scars are firm pink shiny plaques within the confines of an established scar; keloids grow bulbously beyond the original scar and can often occur at piercing sites
- Sebaceous hyperplasia: Pink to orange doughnut-shaped small papules on the face of adults
- Digital mucous cyst: Tense shiny nodule near DIP, representing joint fluid leakage because of osteoarthritis/injury; drainage of the viscous fluid can temporarily relieve pressure but ortho/hand surgeon intervention is often needed to ultimately prevent recurrence

6.12 PRURITUS

Overview
- Pruritus
  - Transmitted via unmyelinated C and A delta fibers
  - Skin and cornea only tissues that itch
  - Histamine #1 mediator
  - Others include papain, trypsin, serotonin, bradykinin, kallidin, kallikrein, substance P, VIP
  - Prostaglandins exaggerate existing itch
  - Opiates have both central and peripheral itch-producing action

Conditions that Cause Pruritus
- Chronic renal disease
  - 80% of those on dialysis
    - Secondary hyperparathyroidism is an occasional cause of uremic pruritus
  - Increased population of mast cells in skin
  - Tx
    - Emollients, antihistamines ineffective
    - UV phototherapy may benefit
- Cholestasis
  - High level of bile salts
  - Tx: Cholestyramine causes symptomatic improvement
- Endocrine disease
  - Thyrotoxicosis
    - Increased skin blood flow which raises skin temperature
  - Hypothyroidism
    - Pruritus secondary to the dry skin
  - Postmenopausal pruritus may be generalized or localized, usually in anogenital area
- Malignancy
  - Most common association: Hodgkin's disease and polycythemia vera

- Polycythemia vera
  - 50% have water-induced pruritus
  - Referred to as "bath itch" or aquagenic pruritus
  - May precede development of PV by years
  - Itch is independent of temperature of water
- HIV infection
  - Eosinophilic pustular folliculitis
  - Pruritus of HIV
  - May respond to UVB, PUVA, or dapsone

Workup of Generalized Pruritus

- Physical exam, including pelvic and rectal
- CBC
- Stool for O&P, occult blood
- CXr
- Thyroid, renal, and liver function tests
- Drug history/testing

6.13 URTICARIA/ANGIOEDEMA

Urticaria

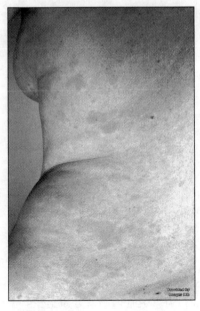

Figure 6.36: Urticaria

- Individual lesions called wheals; may have pale centers (not dusky, so not targetoid)
  - By definition lesions should last <24-hours
    - Ask the patient: "Do they move around?"
- Note: Chronic urticaria defined as ≥6 weeks
- Urticaria may be a disease spectrum with depth of swelling causing urticaria, angioedema (deeper in dermis/subq), or both
- Type I hypersensitivity
- Often caused by: Idiopathic, drug, food, infection (GAS, viral, parasites)

- Primary effector cell = mast cell
  - Pre-formed mediators = histamine, heparin, tryptase, chymase
  - Newly formed mediators = prostaglandins, leukotrienes, PAF
- Types of urticária:
  - Physical urticaria
  - Dermatographism
  - Pressure urticaria
  - Cold urticaria
  - Solar urticaria

Angioedema

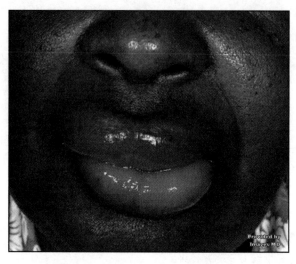

Figure 6.37 Angioedema

- Look for stridor, GI/respiratory symptom
- Can be caused by ACE inhibitors at any time
- C1 esterase inhibitor deficiency
  - Never causes urticaria
  - Screen for with C4 level
  - Can be inherited or acquired
  - Treat with danazol
- Acquired
  - See in lymphoproliferative and rheumatological disease
  - Serum C1q decreased
  - C2 and C4 are decreased in both forms
  - Treatment
    - Androgen therapy: Danazol or stanozolol as prevention
    - Fresh frozen plasma or C1INH should be given in acute attacks
- Diagnosis review
  - Screen with C3 and C4 levels → C4 low, C3 normal in angioedema
  - C1q level low in acquired, but normal in hereditary

Anaphylaxis

- Nonimmunologic urticaria (anaphylactoid drug reaction)
  - Caused by direct mast cell granulation
  - Mnemonic PROMS = polymyxin B, radiocontrast, opioids, muscle relaxants, salicylates/NSAIDs

Urticarial Vasculitis

- Clinically indistinguishable from urticaria, but last >24-hours
- Hypocomplementemic urticarial vasculitis syndrome
  - Defined by low serum complement levels plus presence of anti-C1q precipitin (in 100%), decrease in C1 activity

6.14 COLLAGEN VASCULAR/CONNECTIVE TISSUE DISEASE

*Specifically, most used to refer to spectra of: SLE/RA/dermatomyositis/Sjögren/scleroderma.
**Note: Skin changes non-specific for CVD includes: Raynaud's, non-scarring alopecia, livedo reticularis, pericuticular erythema, telangiectasia, palpable purpura (leukocytoclastic vasculitis) – especially in SLE and RA.

Lupus Erythematosus

Acute

- Types: Malar erythema "butterfly rash," diffuse erythemas, bullous

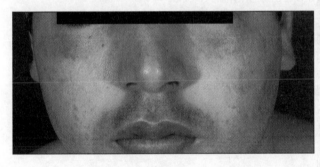

Figure 6.38: Malar erythema of acute lupus erythematosus

- These acute findings are usually associated with SLE, but there is overlap
  - Systemic lupus erythematosus (SLE)
    - Know the 11 criteria, ≥ 4/11 = SLE;
      - 4 skin findings: Malar, discoid, oral ulcers, photosensitivity
      - 2 antibodies: ANA (99% sensitive) and anti-Smith (or anti-dsDNA) (specific)
      - 5 systems: Heme (hemolytic anemia, leukopenia, or thrombocytopenia), renal (proteinuria), neuro (seizures or psychosis), rheum (arthritis), and cards/Pulm (serositis)
    - Note- ANA patterns: Homogeneous (anti-histone), peripheral (anti-dsDNA, SLE with renal dz), speckled, nucleolar (ribosomal RNA, scleroderma), centromeric (Only centromeric is specific: CREST)
    - Lupus band test = DIF shows DEJ IgG deposits in normal, non-sun-exposed skin of SLE

- ○ Drug-induced lupus
  - • Resolves in days to months
  - • Most common: Hydralazine (5%), procainamide (15 to 25% of patients taking the drug), quinidine
  - • Has been reported with minocycline
  - • Anti-histone Ab in 95% - this is positive in 50% of SLE

Subacute

- • Types: Annular (and polycyclic), urticarial, papulosquamous
  - ○ Subacute cutaneous lupus (SCLE)
    - • Strong anti-Ro association, tend to be ANA positive
    - • Can develop Sjögren; half may meet criteria for lupus
    - • Drug-induced by HCTZ, terbinafine (Lamisil) > Ca channel blockers, NSAIDs, griseofulvin, antihistamines
  - ○ Neonatal lupus erythematosus
    - • Risk of 3rd degree heart block (15 to 30%)
    - • Check for Ro (most common in 95%), La, anti-U1-RNP
    - • Mother usually asymptomatic, usually Ro positive (1% risk)
    - • 25% risk of next child developing

Chronic

- • Types: Discoid, panniculitis, hypertrophic/lichenoid
  - ○ Discoid lupus (DLE)

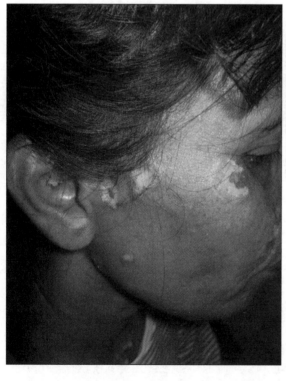

Figure 6.39: Discoid lupus

- • Young adults, women:men 2:1
- • Dull red macules with adherent scales extending into patulous follicles
- • Plugged follicles
- • Patches heal with atrophy, scarring, dyspigmentation, and telangiectasia

- Lupus profundus (panniculitis)
  - Deep dermal and subcutaneous nodules, rubbery-firm, sharply defined, and nontender
  - Upper arms, chest, buttocks, thighs
- Lupus erythematosus tumidus (Tumid lupus)
  - Non-scarring
  - On face/trunk, annular plaques

Pregnancy and SLE
- Miscarriages occur with greater frequency
- LE may worsen, or go into remission during pregnancy
- Fetal death risk increased with anti-cardiolipin or anti-Ro antibodies
- Postpartum period shows the highest risk to the patient

Dermatomyositis

- Clinical signs
  - Gottron's papules = lichenoid papules over MCPs, DIPs, PIPs
  - Gottron's sign = pink/red/purple atrophic or scaling eruption over knuckles, knees, elbows

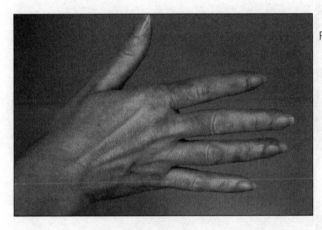

Figure 6.40: Gottron's sign

  - Shawl sign = erythema and scale +/- poikiloderma over shoulders

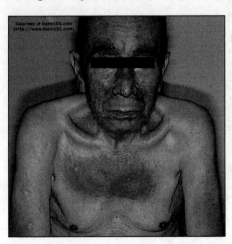

Figure 6.41: Shawl sign

  - On physical exam: Proximal muscle weakness (e.g., cannot lift arms)

- Non-specific: Heliotrope rash (ddx contact dermatitis, trichinosis), poikiloderma, "mechanic's hands," malar erythema
  - Remember: Amyopathic dermatomyositis (atypical case without muscle involvement)
- Frayed cuticular changes in DM = Samitz sign
- Important: r/o underlying malignancy (especially likely if age >50)
  - R/o paraneoplastic syndrome, in women: Ovarian/breast cancer; Men: GI, respiratory cancer
- Antibodies: Anti-Jo-1 (predicts lung involvement), anti-Mi-2 (predicts benign course, less lung involvement), anti-Ku (DM/scleroderma overlap)
- Can see elevated CK and aldolase

Scleroderma

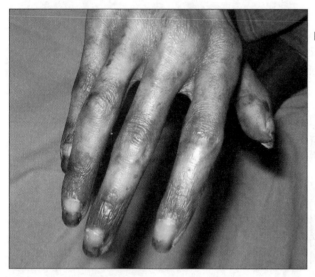

Figure 6.42: Digital tapering of systemic sclerosis

- Localized (morphea)

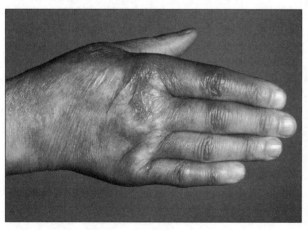

Figure 6.43: Morphea

- Can be associated with anti-ssDNA antibodies
- Melorheostosis = thickening/sclerosis of bones, usually in 1st big toe
- 3 forms: Plaque, linear, generalized
- CREST syndrome
  - Calcinosis, Raynaud's, esophageal dysmotility, sclerodactyly, telangiectasias (matted)

- Anti-centromere ab
- Progressive systemic sclerosis (scleroderma)
- May see CREST findings, plus tightened face, fixed "bird-like" facies, pursed lips, confetti depigmentation, loss of skin creases, digital ulceration, distal pterygium, Raynaud's
- Systemic involvement: Interstitial lung disease, pulmonary HTN, esophageal dysmotility, cardiomyopathy, renal crisis, sicca syndrome
- May have early edematous phase (pitting of digits before sclerosis)
- Anti-Scl-70 Ab
- #1 mortality = lung disease, scleroderma renal crisis

Sjögren

- Keratoconjunctivitis sicca
- Xerostomia
- Rheumatoid arthritis
- More than 90% women
- Vasculitis → palpable purpura
- Patients develop lymphoreticular malignancy such as NHL
- Anti-Ro and La, anti-a-fodrin

Mixed Connective Tissue Disease (MCTD)

- Anti U1-RNP
- Different from overlap of 2 concurrent CTDs

Rheumatoid Arthritis

- Can be associated with vasculitis
- Can be underlying cause of epidermolysis bullosa acquisita
- Rheumatoid nodule

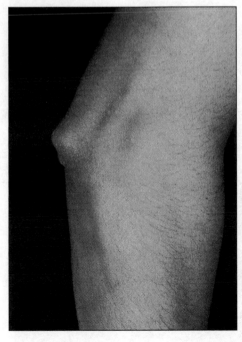

Figure 6.44: Rheumatoid nodule

- Rheumatoid arthritis neutrophilic dermatosis

Relapsing Polychondritis

- On ears, recognized by only affecting cartilage
- Can also affect nose, larynx
- Can see Ab to type II collagen (but found in <50%) - Car-2-lage
- Concern regarding tracheal involvement
- Can be associated with MAGIC syndrome (Mouth And Genital ulcers and Inflamed Cartilage = relapsing polychondritis + Behçet's)

6.15 AUTOIMMUNE BLISTERING DISEASES

Pemphigus Family: Intraepidermal Blisters

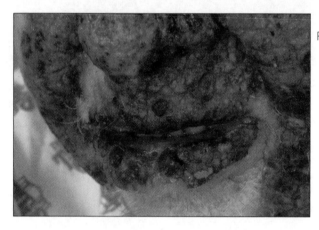

Figure 6.45: Pemphigus vulgaris

- Pemphigus foliaceus - superficial, rarely appreciate intact vesicles. Bran flake-like crust
- Pemphigus vulgaris (mucocutaneous)
- Pemphigus erythematosus (lupus overlap)
- Paraneoplastic (associated with NHL, CLL, thymoma, sarcoma, Castleman)
- Drug induced
    - Thiol-containing drugs: Captopril, penicillamine, thioproline
    - Drugs with disulfide bonds: Gold, pyritinol
    - Drugs that have the potential to release sulfur moieties: Penicillins, piroxicam, cephalosporins
    - Pyrazoline derivatives and enalapril (possibly secondary to an amide group), indomethacin, rifampin

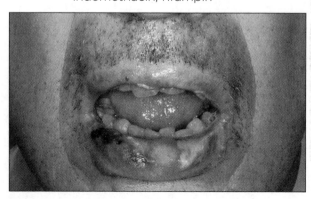

Figure 6.46: Paraneoplastic pemphigus

- Clinical manifestations and diagnosis: Painful pink patches/plaques with erosions (few intact bullae), mucosal ulcerations, bacterial superinfection/sepsis possible
- Diagnosed by skin biopsy/immunofluorescence
- Treatment: Systemic steroids, other immunosuppressants, sometimes rituximab

Subepidermal Blisters

- Clinical manifestations and diagnosis: **Tense**/ruptured bullae, diagnosed by skin biopsy/immunofluorescence
  - Bullous pemphigoid occurs in elderly and can look like urticaria (hives)
  - Dermatitis herpetiformis (DH) extremely pruritic on extremities, often with concurrent celiac disease
  - Linear IgA has necklace-like linked bullae, can be caused by vancomycin
  - Bullous lupus –form of acute lupus
- Treatment: Systemic and topical steroids, dapsone, and gluten-free diet very helpful in DH

6.16 ALOPECIA

Non-scarring Alopecia

- Alopecia areata
  - Genetics
    - High frequency of family history, especially in patients with early onset (37%)
    - Twin concordance = 55% (identical twins)
  - Immunologic factors
    - Major associations: Vitiligo and thyroid disease (10%), with increased prevalence of antithyroid antibodies and thyroid microsomal antibodies in AA
    - Other autoimmune diseases shown to be associated: Pernicious anemia, diabetes, LE, myasthenia gravis, RA, polymyalgia rheumatica, ulcerative colitis
  - Emotional stress
    - May be precipitating factor in some cases
  - Clinical features
    - Pull test may be positive at margins, indicating early disease
    - Usually asymptomatic, but some patients perceive pruritus, tenderness, burning, or pain preceding hair loss
  - PATTERNS: Patchy (most common); reticulated; ophiasis (parietal/temporal/occipital); ophiasis inversus (sisapho – bandlike pattern in fronto parietotemporal scalp)
  - Areata – partial loss of scalp hair
  - Totalis – total loss of scalp hair
  - Universalis – 100% loss on scalp, eyebrows, eyelashes, and rest of body
  - Initial regrowth is white, followed by repigmentation
  - Nail dystrophy (10 to 66%), seen in one, some, or all nails, preceding, coinciding, or occurring after hair disease
    - Pitting with irregular pattern or in organized rows
    - Trachyonychia: Longitudinal striations resulting in sandpaper appearance
    - Red-spotted lunula

- Treatment: Intralesional steroids, topical steroid, systemic steroid, PUVA, topical immunotherapy (e.g., anthralin, diphenylcyclopropenone, squaric acid dibutyl ester), minoxidil

Triangular Alopecia

- Congenital or childhood
- Complete absence of hair or vellus hairs in triangular pattern in the temporal area, frequently bilateral

Androgenetic Alopecia

- AD, polygenetic with variable penetrance
- Progressive miniaturization of hair, increased telogen hairs
- Males – bitemporal, vertex
- Females – preserved anterior hair line, "Christmas-tree" pattern with widened hair part at vertex
- Type II 5-alpha reductase activity in dermal papilla and outer root sheath
- TX: Minoxidil, finasteride, oral contraceptive pills, spironolactone, flutamide, cyproterone acetate, transplant

Trichotillomania

- Compulsive hair pulling, irregular broken hairs within a geometric localized area
- TX: Chlorimipramine, SSRI

Acquired Progressive Kinking

- Post-pubescent male with androgenetic alopecia, gradual curling and darkening of frontal, temporal and auricular regions → progression to androgenetic alopecia
  - Associated with AIDS, retinoids

Syphilis

- Secondary syphilis, 3 to 7% occurrence rate
- "Moth-eaten" – non-scarring with indistinct margins or diffuse alopecia

Telogen Effluvium

- Early and excessive loss of club hairs from the normal resting follicles in the scalp
- Physical stress such as: Surgery, anemia, traction or systemic illness - generally 3 months prior to onset
- Psychological stress
- Endocrine causes such as: Hypo or hyperthyroidism or peri-/postmenopausal states
- Nutritional deficiencies: Biotin, iron, protein (kwashiorkor), zinc, essential fatty acid or calorie deficiency (marasmus or starvation diets)
- Hypervitaminosis A
- Drugs implicated:
  - Amphetamines
  - Aminosalicylic acid
  - Angiotensin-converting enzyme inhibitors
  - Anticoagulants
  - β-blockers
  - Bromocriptine

- ° Carbamazepine
- ° Cimetidine
- ° Danazol
- ° Etretinate
- ° Interferon
- ° Lithium
- ° Oral contraceptives
- ° Valproic acid
- Clinical
  - ° Diffuse loss
  - ° Only rarely involves greater than 50% of the scalp
  - ° Takes 6–12 months for hair density to return to normal therapy

Anagen Effluvium

- ° Frequently seen following administration of cancer chemotherapeutic agents
- ° Stimulus induces the abrupt cessation of mitotic activity in rapidly dividing hair matrix cells; hair shaft thins and then breaks at skin surface
- ° Occurs within days to weeks of the stimulus
- ° Entirely reversible with cessation of drug therapy
- ° Causes
  - Antimetabolites
  - Alkylating agents
  - Mitotic inhibitors
    - – Examples: Doxorubicin, the nitrosoureas, and cyclophosphamide

Alopecia (Scarring)

- Pseudopelade of Brocq

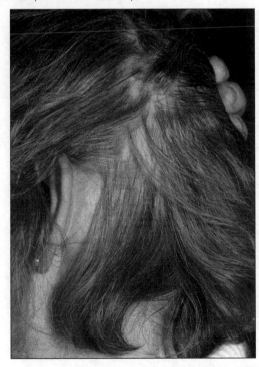

Figure 6.47: Scarring alopecia with Pseudopelade of Brocq

- Alopecia in small patches "foot prints in the snow" to large patches
  - Controversy regarding distinct entity versus end-stage of various scarring alopecias
- Follicular degeneration syndrome
  - Hair loss mostly on vertex in black females +/- history of chemical relaxers
    - Previously known as hot comb alopecia – but can occur without use of hot combs
- Lichen planopilaris

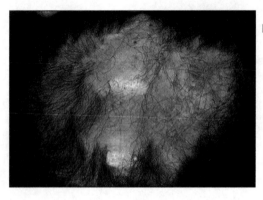

Figure 6.48: Lichen planopilaris

  - Alopecia with perifollicular erythema
- Morphea (en coup de sabre)
  - Linear morphea with linear scarring alopecia of the frontal scalp
  - Parry-Romberg syndrome (linear morphea, progressive facial hemiatrophy, exophthalmos)
- Folliculitis decalvans
  - Inflammation, boggy induration, crust, pustules on scalp
- Dissecting folliculitis (Perifolliculitis Capitis Abscedens et Suffodiens of Hoffman)
  - African American males
  - Deep inflammatory boggy nodules +/- sinus tracts on the occipital region
- Acne keloidalis nuchae
  - African American male
  - Follicular papules and pustules → persistent firm papule or plaque at neck/occipital scalp
- Traction alopecia
  - Prolonged tension on the hair from braiding, ponytails, rolling curlers, twisting with fingers

Other Alopecia
- Meralgia paresthetica
  - May have alopecia of the anesthetic area of the outer thigh
- Hypothyroidism
  - Hair coarse, dry, brittle, and sparse
  - Telogen hairs 3x more prevalent
- Hyperthyroidism
  - Hair becomes extremely fine and sparse
- Alopecia neoplastica
  - Hair loss from metastatic tumors
  - Usually breast carcinoma

6.17 CUTANEOUS MANIFESTATIONS OF INTERNAL DISEASE

Internal Malignancy

- Lung CA →
    - Tripe palms – thick palms with accentuated skin lines and fissures
    - Erythema gyratum repens – pruritic maze-like circular red plaques all over body, migrate daily and rapidly; resolves with treatment of underlying carcinoma
    - Hypertrichosis lanuginosa acquisita – diffuse eruptive downy hair growth starting on face
- Gastrointestinal CA →
    - Sign of Leser-Trélat (gastric adenocarcinoma) – eruptive seborrheic keratoses, often pruritic
    - Tripe palms and severe acanthosis nigricans (gastric adenocarcinoma)
    - Necrolytic migratory erythema (glucagonoma tumor) – psoriasiform eroded eruption with more intertriginous and acral involvement; most patients are metastatic at time of skin diagnosis
- Lymphoproliferative →
    - Paraneoplastic pemphigus (NH lymphoma, CLL, thymoma, Castleman's, sarcoma) – severe mucosal erosions
    - Sweet syndrome (AML) – beefy plaques especially on dorsa of hands
- Genitourinary, breast, or lung CA →
    - Dermatomyositis
        - Sun-exposed scaly pink plaques, heliotrope purple hue around eyes, ragged cuticles, Gottron's papules (pink papules over dorsal hand joints), Gottron's sign (pink papules and nodules over elbows)
        - Proximal muscle weakness
        - Requires CA screening yearly for 5 years after rash appears

Cardiovascular Disease

- Hypertension, venous stasis → stasis dermatitis stasis dermatitis on legs, resembles cellulitis but shows bilateral involvement with background stasis changes; often confused for bilateral cellulitis
- General hyperlipidemia → various types of xanthomas
- Hypertriglyceridemia → eruptive xanthomas
- Metabolic syndrome à acanthosis nigricans, skin tags (*patients with psoriasis carry a higher risk of metabolic syndrome then the general population
- Superior vena cava syndrome → facial edema and dilated veins on skin superior to the heart on the upper chest

Endocrine Disease

- Hypothyroidism →
    - Cool, dry, pale skin, xerosis, hypohidrosis, yellowish hue secondary to carotenemia
    - Generalized myxedema – swollen waxy appearance to skin and lips, broad nose, macroglossia
    - Dry, brittle, coarse, straw-like hair
- Hyperthryoidism →
    - Thyroid acropachy – clubbing of fingers associated with soft tissue swelling and periosteal new bone formation
    - Localized or generalized hypertrichosis, wispy fine hair
    - Thyroid dermopathy (pretibial myxedema) – bilaterally symmetric, non-pitting yellowish-brown to red waxy papules, nodules, and plaques most commonly on lower extremities (but can occur on any area of skin)

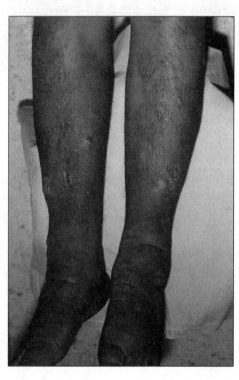

Figure 6.49: Myxedema

- Diabetes mellitus →
    - Acanthosis nigricans, diabetic limited joint mobility (cheiroarthropathy), necrobiosis lipoidica (NL), scleredema, diabetic bullae (bullosis diabeticorum), diabetic dermopathy ("shin spots" or pigmented pretibial papules), eruptive xanthomas, granuloma annulare (generalized and perforating forms), skin tags, perforating dermatoses
    - Can also be associated with other autoimmune skin conditions like vitiligo

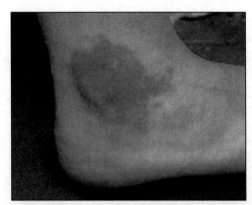

Figure 6.50: Necrobiosis lipoidica

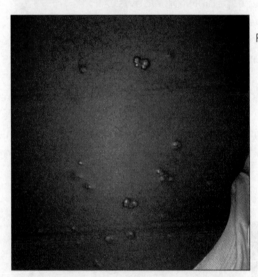

Figure 6.51: Eruptive xanthomas

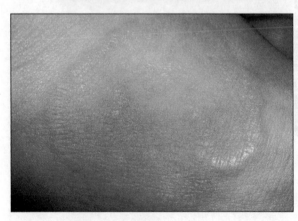

Figure 6.52: Granuloma annulare

Rheumatologic Disease

- Lupus →
    - Photosensitive eruptions – butterfly rash (acute systemic lupus), discoid (scarring especially on face and inside ears), annular (subacute cutaneous lupus)
    - Vasculitis – palpable purpura
    - Alopecia, often scarring
- Dermatomyositis
    - Photosensitive eruption, heliotrope, Gottron's papules, ragged cuticles

Gastrointestinal Disease

- Inflammatory bowel disease
  - Erythema nodosum; ulcerative colitis (UC) > Crohns
  - Cutaneous/metastatic Crohns – vegetative ulcerating plaque with histologic features of Crohns (granulomatous)
  - Pyoderma gangrenosum – ulceration with underminable rolled dusky borders; + pathergy (do not debride); UC > Crohns
  - Gingival hyperplasia and cobblestoning (Crohns)
  - Pyoderma vegetans (UC)
  - Vasculitis/Polyarteritis nodosa (Crohns)
- Celiac disease →
  - Dermatitis herpetiformis – very pruritic, especially on elbows
  - Over 90% of people with the rash have gluten-sensitive enteropathy
  - 15 to 25% celiac patients develop dermatitis herpetiformis
  - Skin disease responds to gluten-free diet (and dapsone)
- Hepatitis C →
  - Porphyria cutanea tarda – sun-exposed papules, bullae, tiny cysts and scars, werewolf-like hair growth on face, 24-hour urine porphyrins is test of choice
  - Lichen planus – purple polygonal pruritic papules, classic area is wrists but can occur anywhere on skin, Wickham striae (can see in mouth), oral erosions (most commonly in setting of Hep C)
  - Necrolytic acral erythema – psoriasiform plaques on dorsa of feet

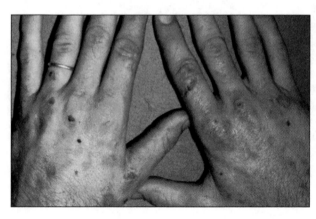

Figure 6.53: Porphyria cutanea tarda

Pulmonary Disease

- Sarcoidosis →
  - Lupus pernio – plum-colored nodules especially on nose, cheeks, and ears
  - Erythema nodosum
- Wegener granulomatosis →
  - Palpable purpura on legs, skin ulcers, erythema nodosum
  - Oral ulcers and gingival hyperplasia (strawberry-like)
- Pulmonary hypertension
  - Clubbing

Figure 6.54: Papular sarcoidosis

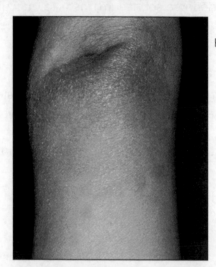

Figure 6.55: Plaque sarcoidosis

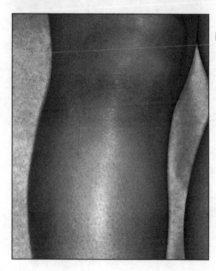

Figure 6.56: Erythema nodosum

Renal Disease

- Renal failure →
    - Pruritus – best treated with light therapy
    - Nephrogenic systemic fibrosis (NSF) – thickening of skin (excluding face), caused by renal insufficiency paired with exposure to MRA with gadolinium contrast

- Calciphylaxis – purple necrotic plaques (the more proximal, the more deadly), caused by calcifications of vessels and thrombosis, often results in severe wounds, infection, and death
- Perforating dermatoses – crusted papules on skin (especially arms) representing extruding material from the body

Neurologic Disease
- Alzheimer's, Parkinson's, stroke → seborrheic dermatitis, increased risk of melanoma
- Neurocutaneous syndromes →
    - Neurofibromatosis – neurofibromas, skin freckling (axilla), café au lait macules, Lisch nodules in iris, scoliosis, seizures
    - Tuberous sclerosis – facial papules (adenoma sebaceum), ash leaf macules (hypopigmented), Shagreen patch (thick leathery truncal plaque), intracranial tubers causing various neurologic symptoms

Pregnancy-related Dermatoses: Usually Late in Pregnancy
- Polymorphous eruption of pregnancy (formerly PUPPP) – pruritic papules starting in striae
- Pemphigoid gestationis – hive-like lesions and bullae starting periumbilically; associated with Grave disease
- Intrahepatic cholestasis of pregnancy – pruritus, abnormal bile acids/cholelithiasis, low maternal K+

Pustular Psoriasis of Pregnancy/Impetigo Herpetiformis
- Late 1st trimester to 3rd trimester
- Clinical
    - Often begins in intertriginous regions and spreads to trunk and extremities
    - Spares face, palms, and soles
    - Erythematous plaque with ring of pustules that enlarges at periphery and erodes or crusts at periphery
    - Mucosa can be involved
    - Onycholysis
- Remits quickly postpartum
- Recurs with subsequent pregnancies, menses, and OCP's
- Fetus at risk for placental insufficiency
- Laboratory
    - Hypocalcemia, leukocytosis, elevated ESR
- Treatment
    - Prednisolone 80 mg/d → decreases mortality risk for mother
    - Treat hypocalcemia
    - May require early delivery

6.18 SELECTED DERMATOLOGIC EMERGENCIES

Stevens-Johnson Syndrome/Toxic Epidermal Necrolysis (TEN)

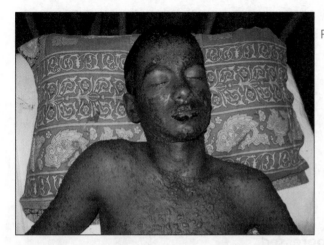

Figure 6.57: Steven Johnson syndrome

- Causes: Medications (sulfa drugs, anticonvulsants, allopurinol, NSAIDs), infections (HSV, mycoplasma)
- Clinical manifestations: Targetoid and eroded pink papules, plaques, and mucosal ulcerations, occurring 1 to 3 weeks after starting offending medication, can progress to full skin sloughing (TEN)/death
- Diagnosis and management: Clinical features (+/- skin biopsy), treatment = avoidance triggers, prompt supportive therapy to avert infection and shock

DRESS (Drug Reaction With Systemic Symptoms and Eosinophilia)

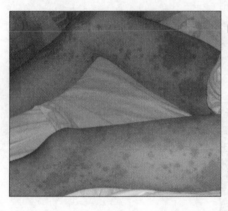

Figure 6.58: Morbilliform eruption of DRESS

- Causes: Medications (anticonvulsants, antibiotics, allopurinol); valproic acid safe
- Clinical manifestations: Rapidly-progressive drug rash and facial edema, usually within 2 to 8 weeks of drug exposure, recurs quickly with re-exposure
- Diagnosis and management: Clinical features and eosinophilia/possible liver and renal dysfunction, treatment = prompt drug withdrawal, long taper of steroid usually required

Erythroderma

- Causes: Psoriasis, atopic dermatitis, drug eruption, cutaneous lymphoma, paraneoplastic, idiopathic
- Clinical manifestations: Diffusely erythematous scaly skin, sometimes with ectropion
- Diagnosis and management: Clinical history and skin biopsy; treatment = etiology-based, often topical and systemic steroids and antihistamines, IV fluids

6.19 SPECIAL POPULATIONS

Skin in Elderly Patients

- Common clinical problems of aging skin: Photoaging (wrinkles, lentigines, actinic purpura), seborrheic keratoses, actinic keratoses, xerosis (dry skin), pruritus, brittle hair and nails, pattern hair loss

Dermatologic Diseases in the Immunosuppressed

- HIV: Pruritus, eosinophilic folliculitis, facial lipoatrophy (see Figure on nasolabial lipoatrophy), Kaposi sarcoma (see Figure on Kaposi's sarcoma), infection (diffuse molluscum, warts, herpes, scabies, oral hairy leukoplakia/EBV)

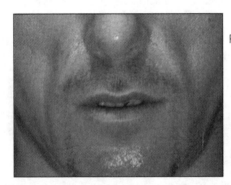

Figure 6.59: Nasolabial lipoatrophy

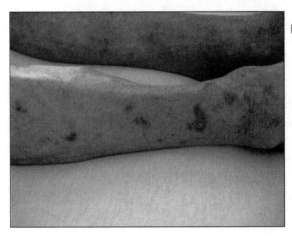

Figure 6.60: Kaposi's sarcoma

- Transplant patients: Skin cancer (highest risk is for squamous cell carcinoma – 36 fold), graft-versus host disease (GVHD), disseminated infections

6.20 HIGH YIELD

Childhood Viral Exanthems

- First disease – Rubeola/measles – Paramyxovirus
- Second disease – Scarlet fever – Streptococcus (not viral)
- Third disease – Rubella – Togavirus
- Fourth disease – Duke's disease – not specific
- Fifth disease – Erythema infectiosum – Parvovirus B19
- Sixth disease – Roseola/Exanthem subitum – HHV-6/7

Human Herpes Viruses

- HHV-1 = HSV-1
- HHV-2 = HSV-2
- HHV-3 = VZV
- HHV-4 = EBV
- HHV-5 = CMV
- HHV-6 = related to pityriasis rosea and roseola, DRESS
- HHV-7 = related to pityriasis rosea and roseola, DRESS
- HHV-8 = related to Kaposi's sarcoma, Castleman disease, primary effusion lymphoma
- Alpha = HHV-1,2,3 (herpes ones)
- Beta = HHV-5,6,7 (CMV, roseola)
- Gamma = HHV-4 and 8 (oncogenic ones)

Causes of Gingival Hyperplasia

- Drugs: Phenytoin, Ca channel blockers, cyclosporine
- Diseases: AML, sarcoid, Wegener's, scurvy, pregnancy, upper airway disease

HCV Skin Associations

(By direct effect and as consequence of associated hepatic damage)
- Cutaneous necrotizing vasculitis (as in type II cryoglobulinemia), usually presents with palpable purpura, can see livedo reticularis, urticaria
- Porphyria cutanea tarda (may have HCV association)
- Lichen planus – stronger association with mucosal/ulcerative LP
- Cutaneous B-cell lymphoma
- Xerostomia
- Erythema multiforme (possibly)
- Pruritus (in 15% of patients with HCV)
- Necrolytic Acral Erythema

HIV Skin Associations

- Exuberant seborrheic dermatitis
- Kaposi's sarcoma
- Molluscum contagiosum (giant, diffuse)
- HIV-associated eosinophilic pustular folliculitis
- Diffuse tinea corporis
- Herpes zoster (and disseminated zoster)
- Lipodystrophy – associated with protease inhibitors (specifically indinavir)
- Bacillary angiomatosis

- TB and atypical mycobacteria (esp. MAC)
- Cryptococcosis
- Toxoplasmosis
- Reactive arthritis (psoriasiform)
- Diffuse verruca vulgaris/ condyloma acuminata
- Pruritus

Can also see: Acquired ichthyosis, drug reactions, and psoriasis

Dermatology Conditions Associated With Diabetes

- Acanthosis nigricans
- Diabetic dermopathy ("shin spots")
- Necrobiosis lipoidica (NLD)
- Scleredema
- Granuloma annulare
- Yellow skin (carotenodermia)
- Diabetic bullae (bullous diabeticorum)
- Acrochordon
- Necrotizing fasciitis
- Malignant external otitis
- Erythrasma
- Mucormycosis

Diseases With Body Lice as a Vector

- Body lice = *Pediculus humanus var. corporis*
- Louse-borne epidemic typhus (*Rickettsia prowazekii*)
- Relapsing fever (*Borrelia recurrentis*)
- Trench fever (*Bartonella quintana*)

Types of Cutaneous TB

- From external exposure:
    - Primary inoculation
    - Tuberculosis verrucosa cútis
    - Tuberculosis cutis orificialis (orificial TB)
- From hematogenous spread:
    - Lupus vulgaris
    - Miliary tuberculosis
- From direct extension:
    - Scrofuloderma
- Reactive eruptions to TB (tuberculid eruptions):
    - Papulonecrotic tuberculid
    - Lichen scrofulosorum
        - Erythema induratum

Causes of Urticaria

Mnemonic = Mr. Hives still seeks drugs and graft
- Viral (MR. HIVES) = <u>M</u>easles, <u>R</u>ubella, <u>H</u>epatitis, <u>I</u>nfectious mono (including EBV, CMV, HIV), <u>V</u>iral other, <u>E</u>. infectiosum/<u>S</u>ubitum

- Bacterial (STILL) = Scarlet fever, Toxic shock/strep, Infectious bacterial other (rose spots, salmonella), Lyme, Lues (syphilis)
- Inflammatory (SEEKS) = SLE, Erythema marginatum, Erythema multiforme, Kawasaki's, Still's/serum sickness

I's of Urticaria
- Infection (viral)
- Iatrogenic
- Inherited
- Immunologic
- Idiopathic
- Ingestion (food, drug)
- Injection
- Inhalation
- Infestation
- Physical causes (pressure, cold)

Dermatome Review
- Thumb = C6
- Nipple = T4
- Umbilicus = T10
- Top of feet = L5
- Bottom of feet = S1

Etiologies of Vasculitis (CTD SING)
- CTD (SLE, RA)
- Thrombotic (TTP, DIC, septic emboli, HSP, cryo)
- Drugs (including serum sickness)
- Syndromes (Schnitzler's, Muckle-Wells, Finklestein's disease)
- Infection (HCV, HBV, Strep, GC, HIV)
- Neoplasms (Hodgkin's, multiple myeloma, leukemia)
- Granulomatous/Inflammatory (Churg-Strauss, Wegener's, MPA)

REFERENCES & SUGGESTED READINGS

1. Freedberg IM, Eisen AZ, Wolff K, et al., eds. Fitzpatrick's dermatology in general medicine. 5th ed. New York: McGraw-Hill, Health Professions Division, 1999.

2. Ingham E et al. Proinflammatory levels of interleukin-1 alpha-like bioactivity are present in the majority of open comedones in acne vulgaris. *J Invest Dermatol*. 1992; 98: 895-901.

3. Kim J et al. Activation of toll-like receptor 2 in acne triggers inflammatory cytokine responses. *J Immunol*. 2002; 169:1535-1541.

4. Andrews' diseases of the skin, 9th ed. Philadelphia: WB Saunders, 2000.

5. Goldstein SM and Wintroub BU, Adverse cutaneous reactions to medications. Baltimore: Williams and Wilkins, 1996; 55-57.

6. Wolverton, SE. Comprehensive dermatologic drug therapy. Philadelphia: WB Saunders, 2001.

7. Wolverton, SE. Comprehensive dermatologic drug therapy. Philadelphia: WB Saunders, 2001.

8. Elder D et al. Lever's histopathology of the skin, 8th ed. Philadelphia: Lipincott Raven, 2001; 295.

9. Webster G Fetal. Suppression of polymorphonuclear leukocytechemoactic factor production in Propionibacterium acnes by subminimal inhibitory concentrations of tetracycline, ampicillin, minocycline and erythromycin. Antimicrob agents chemother. 1982; 21:770-772.

10. Wolverton,SE.Comprehensivedermatologicdrugtherapy.Philadelphia:WBSaunders,2001.

11. Dermatology in General Medicine, 5th Edition. New York, McGraw-Hill,1999.

12. Andrews' Diseases of the Skin, 9th Edition. Philadelphia:WB Saunders,2000.

13. http://www.cdc.gov/lyme/

14. http://www.cdc.gov/rmsf/

15. http://www.cdc.gov/parasites/lice/

16. Goldsmith L, et al. Fitzpatrick's Dermatology in General Medicine 8e, New York: McGraw Hill, 2012.

17. Rigopoulos D, et al. Skin signs of systemic diseases. *Clin Dermatol*. 2011; 29(5): 531-40.

18. Thiers BH, et al. Cutaneous manifestations of internal malignancy. *CA Cancer J Clin*. 2009; 59(2): 73-98.

NOTES

NOTES

INDEX

A

M

NOTES

NOTES

NOTES

NOTES

NOTES

NOTES

NOTES

NOTES

NOTES